Reading MRI of the Prostate

Ananya Panda • Vikas Gulani • Lee Ponsky
Editors

Reading MRI of the Prostate

A Practical Guide

Springer

Editors
Ananya Panda, MD, FRCR
Department of Radiology
Mayo Clinic
Rochester, MN
USA

Vikas Gulani, MD, PhD
Fred Jenner Hodges Professor and Chair
Department of Radiology
University of Michigan
Ann Arbor, MI
USA

Lee Ponsky, MD, FACS
Professor and Chair
Urology Institute
Leo and Charlotte Goldberg Chair of
Advanced Surgical Therapies
Master Clinician in Urologic Oncology
University Hospitals Cleveland
Medical Center
Case Western Reserve University
School of Medicine
Cleveland, OH
USA

ISBN 978-3-319-99355-3 ISBN 978-3-319-99357-7 (eBook)
https://doi.org/10.1007/978-3-319-99357-7

This Springer imprint is published by the registered company Springer Nature Switzerland AG
The registered company address is: Gewerbestrasse 11, 6330 Cham, Switzerland

Lee would like to dedicate this book to his wife Monica and their three children, Ilan, Eric, and Maiya who always remind him what is most important in life.

Contents

Contributors

Laura Bukavina, MD Urology Institute, University Hospitals Cleveland Medical Center, Cleveland, OH, USA

Case Western Reserve University School of Medicine, Cleveland, OH, USA

Christina Buzzy, PhD Urology Institute, University Hospitals Cleveland Medical Center, Cleveland, OH, USA

Case Western Reserve University School of Medicine, Cleveland, OH, USA

Vikas Gulani, MD, PhD Fred Jenner Hodges Professor and Chair, Department of Radiology, University of Michigan, Ann Arbor, MI, USA

Amr Mahran, MD Urology Institute, University Hospitals Cleveland Medical Center, Cleveland, OH, USA

Case Western Reserve University School of Medicine, Cleveland, OH, USA

Kirtishri Mishra, MD Urology Institute, University Hospitals Cleveland Medical Center, Cleveland, OH, USA

Case Western Reserve University School of Medicine, Cleveland, OH, USA

Verena Obmann, MD Department of Diagnostic, Interventional and Pediatric Radiology (DIPR), Inselspital, Bern University Hospital, University of Bern, Bern, Switzerland

Ananya Panda, MD, FRCR Department of Radiology, Mayo Clinic, Rochester, MN, USA

Lee Ponsky, MD, FACS Professor and Chair, Urology Institute, Leo and Charlotte Goldberg Chair of Advanced Surgical Therapies, Master Clinician in Urologic Oncology, University Hospitals Cleveland Medical Center, Case Western Reserve University School of Medicine, Cleveland, OH, USA

About the Book

This book is intended to serve as a source for urologists and radiologists who want to develop an understanding of MRI of the prostate. As with any developing technology, there will continue to be advancements and innovations in the field. However, a fundamental understanding of MRI of the prostate presented in this book from both a radiology and urology perspective will help to serve as a foundation for understanding the current state and, to build upon for future developments and clinical integration of prostate imaging.

About the Editors

Ananya Panda is a clincial fellow in Nuclear Radiology, with a propsective academic appointment of Assistant Professor at the Mayo Clinic, Rochester. She completed her primary Radiology Residency from All India Institute of Medical Sciences (AIIMS), New Delhi, India in 2013. Thereafter, she spent three years at AIIMS as a senior resident invested in patient care and academic teaching. She subsequently pursued a two-year postdoctoral fellowship in Body MRI at Case Western Reserve University, Cleveland, Ohio working on the clinical translation of quantitative MRI and exploring the utility of multiparametric imaging, with a focus on prostate imaging. She is the recipient of several awards including Radiology Society of North America (RSNA) Trainee Research Awards in 2018 and 2019 for research work in prostate cancer and pancreatic cancer and the Gold Medal for the Best Radiology Resident in 2014. She was admitted as a Fellow of the Royal College of Radiology (UK) in 2018. Her clinical interests lie in exploring multiparametric and hybrid imaging for emerging clinical applications in body imaging, oncology and nuclear radiology.

Vikas Gulani is the Chair and Fred J. Hodges Professor of Radiology at the University of Michigan, Ann Arbor. Dr. Gulani received his B.S. in Chemical Engineering at UCLA. He then moved to the University of Illinois at Urbana-Champaign, completing his Ph.D. in Physiology under Prof. Paul C. Lauterbur, the winner of the 2003 Nobel Prize for Medicine or Physiology for the invention of Magnetic Resonance Imaging (MRI). After his MD also at Illinois, he completed a Diagnostic Radiology residency and fellowship in Body MRI at the University of Michigan. During residency, he spent a year at the University of Würzburg in Germany, working as a research postdoctoral fellow in the Department of Physics. He joined the faculty in the Department of Radiology at Case Western Reserve University and University Hospitals after training, and was the Joseph T. Wearn Professor, Professor of Radiology, Biomedical Engineering, and Urology, a member of the Case Comprehensive Cancer Center, and the Director of MRI for the University Hospitals system. His clinical interests include all abdominal/pelvic imaging, but particularly prostate, liver, and renal MRI and MR angiography. His past and present research interests in MRI include MR fingerprinting and quantitative MRI, parallel imaging and rapid acquisitions, diffusion tensor imaging and diffusion anisotropy, perfusion MRI, MR microscopy, and body MRI. His most recent work includes the invention with his collaborators of the MR fingerprinting technology, and he has spearheaded the effort to bring this work to clinical fruition, bringing together his engineering and clinical knowledge and scientific and industry collaborations. In prostate imaging, he has worked on the clinical translation of MR fingerprinting, development of an all-quantitative MRI exam, a rapid screening protocol, and in-bore prostate biopsies. As Chair, his primary goal is to build a compassionate workplace that strives toward excellence.

Lee Ponsky attended University of Rochester as an undergraduate and then Case Western Reserve University School of Medicine. He began his training at the Cleveland Clinic and completed his residency and extended his training to do a research fellowship in urologic oncology, followed by an additional fellowship in Advanced Urologic Laparoscopy and Endourology.

In 2005, Lee joined the faculty at University Hospitals, Case Western Reserve University School of Medicine, and is currently the Chairman of the Department of Urology and Director of the Urology Institute. He is a Professor of Urology and holds the Leo and Charlotte Goldberg Chair in Advanced Surgical Therapies and a Master Clinician in Urologic Oncology. He has over 100 publications and has been invited as a visiting professor at numerous national and international conferences and institutions. Lee is the co-principal investigator on an NIH RO1 grant. He is the Editor-in-Chief of a textbook on Robotic Radiosurgery and has authored more than 12 textbook chapters. Lee recently founded IOIO Studio, a tattoo removal, and MediSpa Studio and Walden Medical, a medical device company.

Lee has received numerous accolades for his medical contributions as well as for his role as the founder of MedWish International in 1993. MedWish is a not-for-profit organization that saves lives and the environment by repurposing discarded medical supplies and equipment to provide humanitarian aid in developing countries. His recognitions include U.S. Congressional Recognition, Crain's Forty under Forty, as one of Northeast Ohio's most influential people under the age of 40, Cleveland Upstander: Portraits of Courage, the recipient of the Golden Doc Award, from the Arnold P. Gold Foundation, and received the Rescuer of Humanity Award from Project Love, which recognizes and honors an individual or an organization of national or international stature, which has chosen to use their leadership beyond professional or institutional requirements to positively change the course of humanity. He has also been recognized by the Manhattan Institute in New York with the Richard Cornuelle Award for Social Entrepreneurship, for originating and effectively implemented a new nonprofit organization providing direct services to those in need. In 2011, he was recognized by Smart Business as the nonprofit board executive of the year and also received the University Hospitals Case Medical Center, Urology Institute Faculty Teaching Award from his students and residents, for recognition of outstanding commitment and efforts to student and resident teaching. In 2019, he received the Champion of Integrity Award by the Better Business Bureau for consistently displaying an aggressive commitment to ethical, honest, and fair business practices.

Lee also serves as a founding board member of the nonprofit MedWorks, which provides free healthcare to the uninsured and underinsured.

1 Introduction

Ananya Panda, Vikas Gulani, and Lee Ponsky

Magnetic Resonance Imaging (MRI) currently plays a vital role in evaluation of the prostate gland. Conventional anatomic MRI combined with functional imaging allows multi-parametric MRI (mpMRI) evaluation of the prostate that has become the standard in evaluating this organ by imaging. Recently, results from multiple important prostate MRI trials have provided increasing evidence for an MRI-guided strategy in the management of prostate cancer. Trials such as PROstate MR Imaging Study (PROMIS) [1], and later Prostate Evaluation for Clinically Important disease (PRECISION) [2] provided critical data supporting such a strategy. In this book, we review the rationale behind the mpMRI approach, and provide a simple pictorial guide to approaching MRI of the prostate.

Chapters have been organized to serve as building blocks to understanding, acquiring and interpreting prostate MRIs. Thus we begin with normal MR anatomy, proceed to a typical mpMRI protocol and then discuss prostate MR interpretation and reporting under the consensus Prostate Imaging, Reporting and Data System (PI-RADS)- version 2 and 2.1 guidelines released in 2015 and 2019 respectively [3, 4]. Subsequent chapters deal with MR appearances of atypical locations of

A. Panda
Department of Radiology, Mayo Clinic, Rochester, MN, USA
e-mail: panda.ananya@mayo.edu

V. Gulani (✉)
Fred Jenner Hodges Professor and Chair, Department of Radiology,
University of Michigan, Ann Arbor, MI, USA
e-mail: vikasgulani@med.umich.edu

L. Ponsky
Professor and Chair, Urology Institute, Leo and Charlotte Goldberg
Chair of Advanced Surgical Therapies, Master Clinician in Urologic Oncology,
University Hospitals Cleveland Medical Center, Case Western Reserve
University School of Medicine, Cleveland, OH, USA
e-mail: Lee.Ponsky@UHhospitals.org

A. Panda et al. (eds.), *Reading MRI of the Prostate*,
https://doi.org/10.1007/978-3-319-99357-7_1

prostate cancer and common tumor mimics. Further more, we also briefly discuss the evolving role of biparametric MRI in prostate cancer screening, the role of MRI in active surveillance and the potential utility of quantitative MRI in prostate imaging.

While no book can ever be totally comprehensive, we hope that that this book serves as a useful guide for reading MRI of the prostate for both clinicians and radiologists.

References

1. Ahmed HU, Bosaily AE-S, Brown LC, et al. Diagnostic accuracy of multi-parametric MRI and TRUS biopsy in prostate cancer (PROMIS): a paired validating confirmatory study. Lancet. 2017;389(10071):815–22.
2. Kasivisvanathan V, Rannikko AS, Borghi M, et al. MRI-targeted or standard biopsy for prostate-cancer diagnosis. N Engl J Med. 2018;378(19):1767–77.
3. Barentsz JO, Weinreb JC, Verma S, et al. Synopsis of the PI-RADS v2 guidelines for multiparametric prostate magnetic resonance imaging and recommendations for use. Eur Urol. 2016;69(1):41–9.
4. Turkbey B, Rosenkrantz AB, Haider MA, et al. Prostate imaging reporting and data system version 2.1: 2019 update of prostate imaging reporting and data system version 2. Eur Urol. 2019;76(3):340–51.

Normal Anatomy of Prostate

2

Ananya Panda and Vikas Gulani

T1 and T2 relaxation times are MR-specific intrinsic properties of tissue. These characteristic times affect all MR images, and MR images are made intentionally more sensitive to differences in T1 or T2 relaxation times, or in other words, are T1 or T2 "weighted." Prostate anatomy is best depicted on high resolution, small field of view, T2 weighted images. Using three-plane T2 weighted images in sagittal, coronal and axial planes, it is possible to visualize the different zones of prostate as described by McNeal [1].

In the coronal plane, the prostate is a walnut shaped organ, broader at the top and narrowing down inferiorly. The prostate is divided cranio-caudally into the base, mid-gland and apex, each comprising one-third of the gland. The base of the prostate borders the urinary bladder and the apex is at the caudal aspect of the prostate. The seminal vesicles are located posterior to the prostate. The ejaculatory ducts course in posterior part of the prostate to insert into prostatic urethra at the level of verumontanum [2] (Fig. 2.1).

Anatomically, the prostate has been divided on imaging into the peripheral zone (PZ), transition zone (TZ), central zone (CZ) and anterior fibromuscular stroma (AFMS). The urethra and the verumontanum are used as key reference landmarks to separate various zones of prostate [3]. In the sagittal plane, the urethra has an oblique course with a 35-degree anterior angulation midway through the base and apex of the prostate, dividing the prostatic urethra into proximal and distal parts (Fig. 2.2). The proximal prostatic urethra is related to the transition zone, which surrounds it both anteriorly and posteriorly. The central zone lies behind the transition

A. Panda
Department of Radiology, Mayo Clinic, Rochester, MN, USA
e-mail: panda.ananya@mayo.edu

V. Gulani (✉)
Fred Jenner Hodges Professor and Chair, Department of Radiology, University of Michigan, Ann Arbor, MI, USA
e-mail: vikasgulani@med.umich.edu

A. Panda et al. (eds.), *Reading MRI of the Prostate*,
https://doi.org/10.1007/978-3-319-99357-7_2

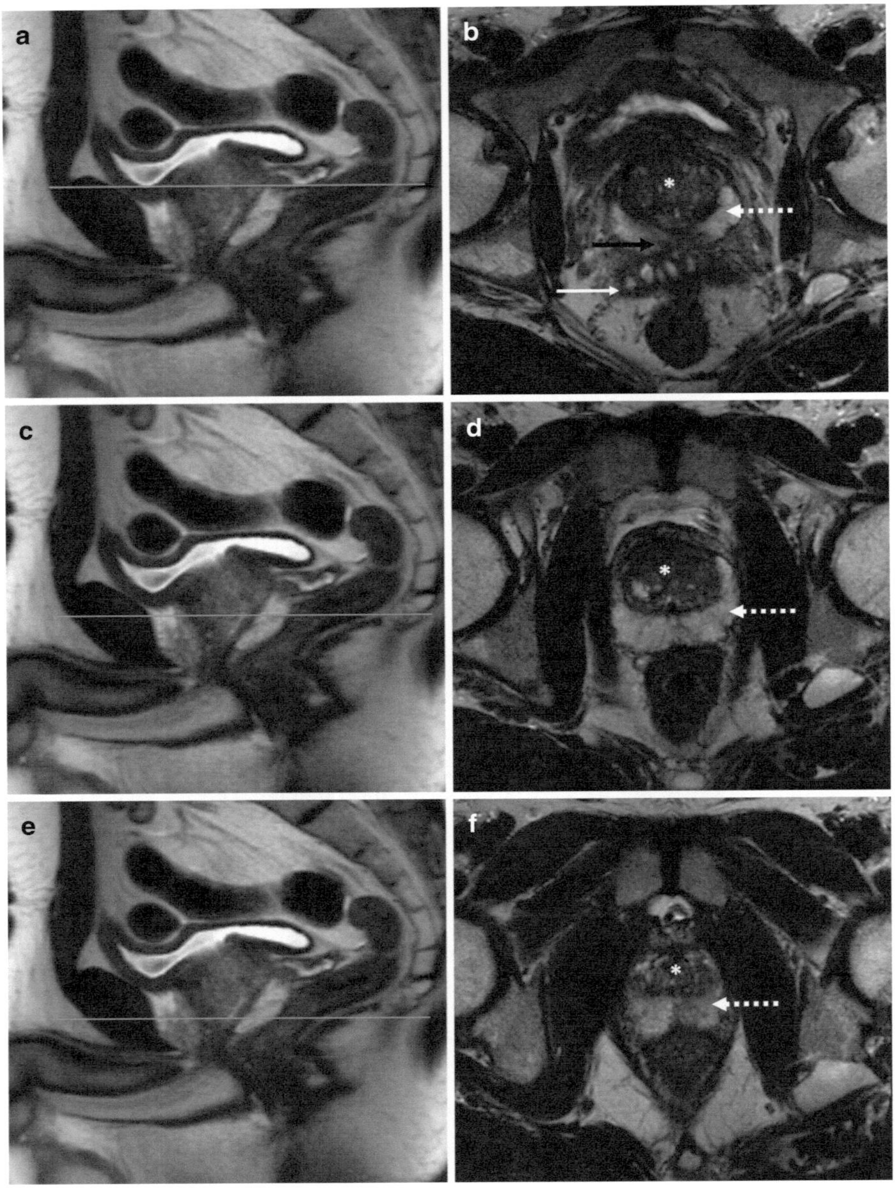

Fig. 2.1 T2 weighted sagittal and axial sections showing the base (**a**, **b**), mid-gland (**c**, **d**) and apex (**e**, **f**) of the prostate. At all three levels, the normal peripheral zone (white dotted arrow) is bright, while the transition zone has a heterogeneous appearance (asterisk). The base is also contiguous with seminal vesicles (white arrow, **b**) and the central zone (black arrow, **b**)

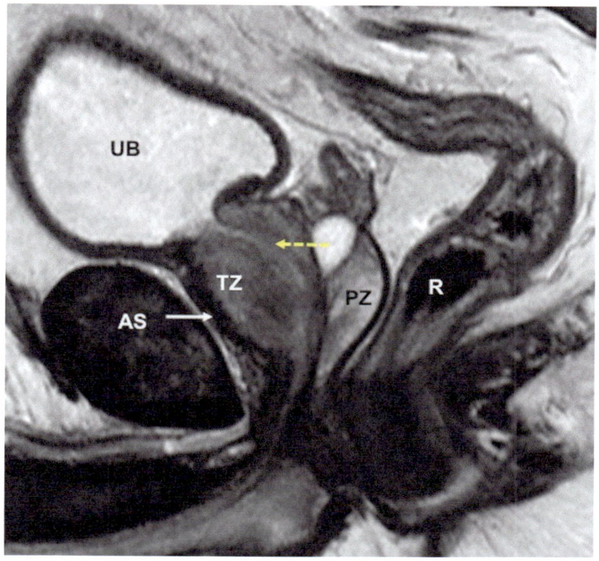

Fig. 2.2 Sagittal T2 weighted image shows oblique course of urethra (yellow dotted arrow) surrounded by transition zone (TZ). The peripheral zone (PZ) is seen below and behind the transition zone. The anterior stroma (AS) is seen as a dark band anteriorly. The rectum (R) is located behind the prostate while urinary bladder (UB) sits atop the prostate

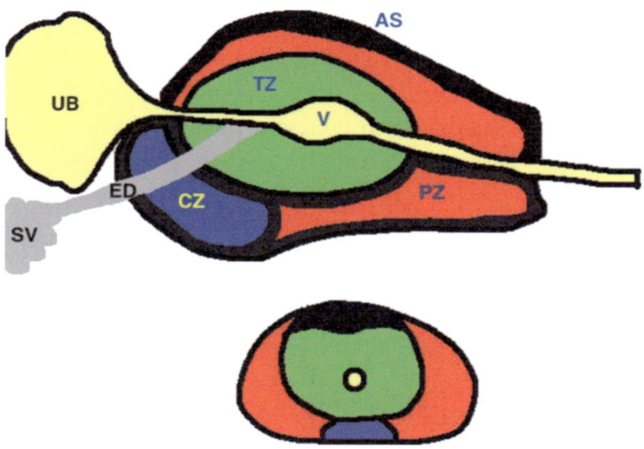

Fig. 2.3 Sagittal and transverse line diagrams of the prostate show the different anatomic regions of prostate and their relationships to each other. *PZ* peripheral zone, *TZ* transition zone, *SV* seminal vesicles, *ED* ejaculatory ducts, UB urinary bladder, *AS* anterior stroma, urethra is shown in yellow with verumontanum (V) in the center

zone and superior to verumontanum and is intimately related to the ejaculatory ducts. The peripheral zone subtends both the central zone and the transition zone and forms a major part of the midgland and apex of the prostate, such that the distal prostatic urethra is almost entirely surrounded by the peripheral zone. The anterior fibromuscular stroma hangs anteriorly like a curtain, covering the anterior aspect of transition zone [4] (Fig. 2.3).

In younger men (less than 35–40 years of age) the transition zone is just a small disk of tissue surrounding the proximal prostatic urethra while central zone is much more prominent forming nearly 25% of the gland [4]. With age, the transition zone undergoes significant nodular hypertrophy, flattening the central zone and displacing it superiorly towards to the base. The hypertrophied transition zone also forms the median lobe of prostate, which protrudes into the bladder neck. While earlier MR descriptions tended to clump the transition zone and central zone together into a "central gland", it is now known that transition zone and central zone can be distinguished from each other on high-resolution T2 weighted images [5].

Normal MR Appearances of Various Zones

Peripheral Zone The normal peripheral zone has homogeneous high signal intensity on T2 weighted images. In the axial section, it forms the lateral and outer parts of the prostate, increasing in bulk towards mid-gland and apex. The high signal of the peripheral zone has been attributed to the glandular composition of the peripheral zone and the loose arrangement of muscle fibers in the peripheral zone as compared to the central zone. The peripheral zone is also the most common site of prostate cancer with 70% of prostate cancers arising from it [6] (Fig. 2.1b, d, f).

Central Zone The normal central zone is seen only in the superior half of prostate and lies behind the proximal prostatic urethra. It is best visualized in the coronal plane and appears to have a homogeneously low to intermediate signal intensity on T2 weighted images. The normal central zone is bilaterally symmetrical and ejaculatory ducts can be seen coursing through it (Fig. 2.4). With age, the central zone undergoes progressive atrophy, is displaced superiorly towards the base, and may

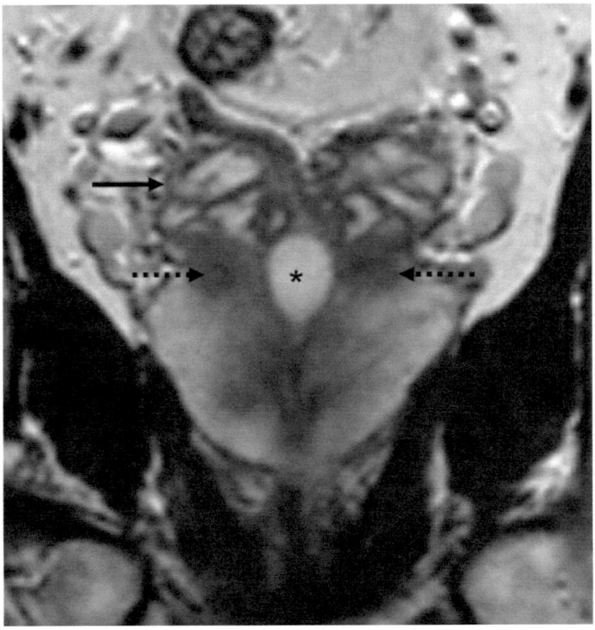

Fig. 2.4 Coronal T2 weighted image show the central gland at the base of the prostate (dotted arrows) intimately associated with the seminal vesicles (black arrow) and surrounded by the bright peripheral zone. The central oval-shaped bright structure ("asterisk") is an incidentally detected prostatic utricle cyst (an embryologic remnant)

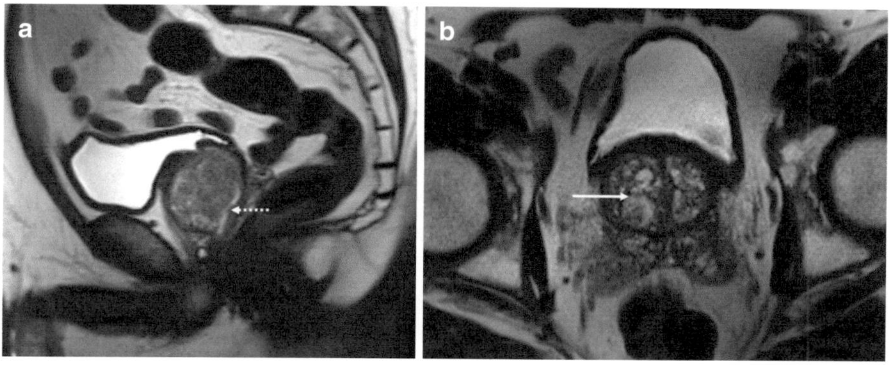

Fig. 2.5 T2 weighted sagittal and axial images show hypertrophied transition zone pushing the urethra (dotted arrow, **a**) posteriorly and causing bladder outlet obstruction. Also note the heterogeneous signal intensity and multiple hyperplastic nodules (arrow, **b**)

have more heterogeneous intermediate signal intensity [5]. The low-intermediate signal intensity in the central zone has been attributed to the presence of stroma and more tightly packed muscle fibers [3]. While the central zone is an uncommon site of prostate cancer with 1–5% of all prostate cancers arising from it, recognition of normal appearances of central zone is important as it can often be misinterpreted as cancer due to its configuration and low signal intensity [7].

Transition Zone The normal transition zone also has intermediate-low signal intensity due to the high proportion of stroma, smooth muscle fibers and periurethral glands associated with the transition zone. With age, the transition zone appears more heterogeneous, with multiple well-circumscribed hyperplastic nodules having intermediate to high signal intensity (Fig. 2.5). About 25% of prostate cancers arise from transition zone and need to be specifically differentiated from stromal hyperplastic nodules.

Anterior Fibromuscular Stroma The normal anterior stroma has homogeneously low signal intensity since it is entirely non-glandular and is composed of stromal and fibrous tissue. Despite its non-glandular composition, up to 8% prostate cancers can be seen in anterior stroma due to contiguous spread from the adjacent peripheral zone or transition zone [8].

Other Relevant Anatomy

Other anatomic structures that can be delineated on MRI include the capsule, the periprostatic neurovascular bundles, urethra, seminal vesicles and ejaculatory ducts. Knowledge of these structures is important for accurate tumor localization and staging.

Capsular structures include the surgical capsule and the outer capsule of the prostate. The surgical capsule is seen as a low-intensity band separating the transition zone and peripheral zone. The outer capsule, though not a specific anatomical structure, is a condensation of fibromuscular tissues around the prostate. It is best seen as a dark band posteriorly and posterolaterally and is well demarcated from the bright signal of periprostatic fat. Any focal irregularity, thickening or discontinuity in the outer capsule is strongly suspicious of extracapsular extension of prostate cancer (Fig. 2.6).

Periprostatic neurovascular bundles (NVB) are best seen posterolaterally at 5 and 7'o clock positions in relation to the prostate, but may also extend more anteriorly. They are seen as low-intensity structures and are especially well-contrasted by the high signal intensity of periprostatic fat (Fig. 2.6). Occasionally normal neurovascular bundles may be mistaken for tumors and thus need to be identified as contiguous tubular structures on non-contrast T1 or T2 weighted images with enhancement after contrast administration [7].

The *urethra and verumontanum* are seen as high intensity structures coursing through the center of prostrate on both axial and coronal planes. The verumontanum is best seen on coronal images and the increased signal intensity is attributed to the mucosal tissue lining the urethra [3].

The *seminal vesicles* are paired lobulated structures that have high signal intensity on T2 weighted images (Fig. 2.1b). The ejaculatory ducts are also seen as small high intensity structures coursing through the central zone. Loss of normal architecture of seminal vesicles, low signal intensity, and enlarged ejaculatory ducts are suspicious for extracapsular extension of cancer.

The *rectum* is seen posterior to the prostate and is separated from it by a distinct fat plane, also called as rectoprostatic angle (Fig. 2.7). Obliteration of this angle and loss of the fat plane indicates extracapsular extension of tumor.

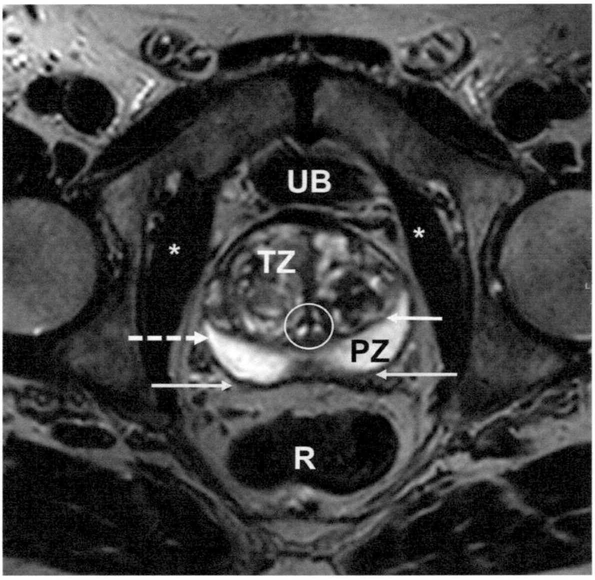

Fig. 2.6 Axial T2 weighted image shows the outer periprostatic capsule (white dotted arrow) and surgical capsule (white solid arrow) between the transition zone (TZ) and surrounding peripheral zone. The urethra is noted in the midline (within circle) and partially compressed by the transition zone. Both neurovascular bundles are seen at 5 and 7 o clock positions (yellow arrows). The rectum (R) and urinary bladder (UB) are seen posterior and anterior to the prostate respectively

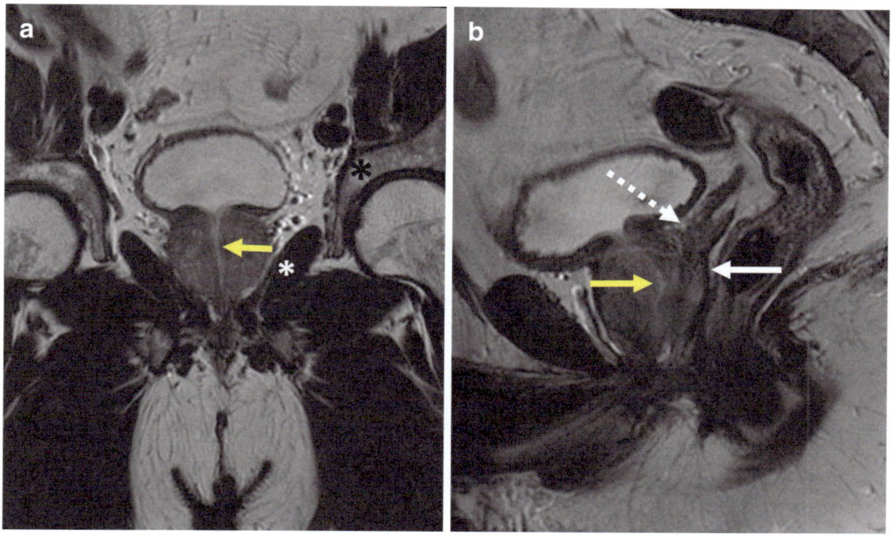

Fig. 2.7 Coronal T2 weighted image (**a**) shows the urethra (yellow arrow), paired levator ani muscles (white asterisk) and pelvic side walls (black asterisk). Sagittal T2 weighted (**b**) image shows the normal acute angle between the seminal vesicle and prostate (dotted arrow) and the normal rectoprostatic fat plane (white arrow)

Checklist for Anatomy (on T2 Weighted Images)

Plane	Structures assessed
Axial (Fig. 2.6)	• Various zones of prostate • Periprostatic structures • Rectum • Urethra • Levator ani muscles • Seminal vesicles
Coronal (Fig. 2.7)	• Central zone • Relationship between central and peripheral zone • Levator ani muscles • Pelvic side walls
Sagittal (Fig. 2.7)	• Angle between seminal vesicles and prostate • Rectoprostatic angle • Interface between prostate and urinary bladder

References

1. McNeal JE. The zonal anatomy of the prostate. Prostate. 1981;2(1):35–49.
2. Hoeks CMA, Barentsz JO, Hambrock T, Yakar D, Somford DM, Heijmink SWTPJ, et al. Prostate cancer: multiparametric MR imaging for detection, localization, and staging. Radiology. 2011;261(1):46–66.

3. Hricak H, Dooms GC, McNeal JE, Mark AS, Marotti M, Avallone A, et al. MR imaging of the prostate gland: normal anatomy. AJR Am J Roentgenol. 1987;148(1):51–8.
4. Selman SH. The McNeal prostate: a review. Urology. 2011;78(6):1224–8.
5. Vargas HA, Akin O, Franiel T, Goldman DA, Udo K, Touijer KA, et al. Normal central zone of the prostate and central zone involvement by prostate cancer: clinical and MR imaging implications. Radiology. 2012;262(3):894–902.
6. McNeal JE, Redwine EA, Freiha FS, Stamey TA. Zonal distribution of prostatic adenocarcinoma. Correlation with histologic pattern and direction of spread. Am J Surg Pathol. 1988;12(12):897–906.
7. Rosenkrantz AB, Taneja SS. Radiologist, be aware: ten pitfalls that confound the interpretation of multiparametric prostate MRI. Am J Roentgenol. 2013;202(1):109–20.
8. Al-Ahmadie HA, Tickoo SK, Olgac S, Gopalan A, Scardino PT, Reuter VE, et al. Anterior-predominant prostatic tumors: zone of origin and pathologic outcomes at radical prostatectomy. Am J Surg Pathol. 2008;32(2):229–35.

Prostate MRI: Technique and Sequences 3

Ananya Panda and Vikas Gulani

With considerable advances in MR technology, MRI has become an established imaging modality for assessment of prostate cancer. In order to standardize prostate MRI exam and reporting, the European Society of Urogenital Radiology (ESUR) established consensus-based guidelines for acquisition, interpretation and structured reporting of prostate MRI known as Prostate Imaging and Reporting Data System (PI-RADS) version 1 (PI-RADS v1) [1]. Thereafter, in 2015, the ESUR and the American College of Radiology (ACR) together released a second version of PI-RADS (PI-RADS v2), which had several important changes [2, 3]. More recently, PI-RADS v2.1 has been released, which further refines MRI protocols and updates evaluation of the transition zone [4].

This chapter elaborates the various MR sequences used in a typical multiparametric MRI (mpMRI) protocol and the minimum technical requirements for an acceptable prostate MR exam, as described in PI-RADS v2.

Pre-procedure Clinical Information

PI-RADS v2 explicitly describes the need for clinicians to provide relevant patient information to radiologists, such as recent serum prostate specific antigen (PSA) levels, PSA history, dates and results of prior prostate biopsy, digital rectal examination results, previous treatment history and family history to ensure more accurate MR reporting.

A. Panda
Department of Radiology, Mayo Clinic, Rochester, MN, USA
e-mail: panda.ananya@mayo.edu

V. Gulani (✉)
Fred Jenner Hodges Professor and Chair, Department of Radiology, University of Michigan, Ann Arbor, MI, USA
e-mail: vikasgulani@med.umich.edu

A. Panda et al. (eds.), *Reading MRI of the Prostate*,
https://doi.org/10.1007/978-3-319-99357-7_3

Timing of MRI Examination

For patients who have had a recent prior prostate biopsy, post-biopsy hemorrhage can confound interpretation of MRI [5, 6]. Hence, PI-RADS v2 recommends waiting for at least 6 weeks after biopsy if MRI is performed for local staging of cancer [7]. However, for detection and characterization of clinically significant cancer, there is no need to delay a mpMRI after a prior biopsy since careful interpretation of anatomic T1 weighted images in combination with diffusion weighted imaging has adequate accuracy for detecting clinically significant cancer, even in the presence of hemorrhage [3, 8].

Patient Preparation

There are no definite consensus guidelines regarding patient preparation for MRI exam. While stool evacuation on the day of MRI is recommended, other invasive methods such as cleansing enemas, suctioning of rectal gas and administration of transrectal ultrasound jelly before MRI are dependent on local institutional policies or may be decided on a case-by-case basis. Similarly using anti-peristaltic agents for mpMRI prostate exam merely adds to the cost of the exam without added benefits. Lastly, PI-RADS v2 no longer recommends abstinence from ejaculation before prostate exam since there is no evidence supporting the benefits of abstinence on accuracy of mpMRI.

Magnetic Field Strength and Coils

Field Strength It is recommended to preferably use 3 T MR scanner for prostate imaging due to higher signal noise ratio (SNR), shorter acquisition time and higher spatial resolution at 3 T compared to 1.5 T [9]. However PI-RADS v2 recognizes that imaging at 1.5 T field strength can also provide acceptable and adequate information using current MR technology. 1.5 T is the first choice when the patient has an implanted device which is MR-conditionally safe at 1.5 T but not at 3 T. Imaging at 1.5 T is also recommended when the patient has a metallic device in the field of view (e.g. bilateral hip prosthesis), which may cause artifacts and affect image quality.

Coils Prostate MRI can be done either with an external/pelvic multichannel array coil or with an endorectal coil. Combining an external phased array coil with an endorectal coil increases SNR at any field strength. A combination of the two may be advantageous when imaging at lower field (1.5 T) for improving resolution for sequences with low SNR.

While endorectal coils provide higher SNR and have utility especially at 1.5 T, they are also more invasive, time–consuming to place and uncomfortable for most patients. The endorectal coil can also potentially deform the gland and induce artifacts. Hence it may be still preferred to use a coil with high number of receiver channels (16 or more) even at 1.5 T instead of an endorectal coil. At 3 T, an array coil is considered to be sufficiently adequate and generally preferred due to patient comfort [10].

Irrespective of the type of coil used, efforts should be taken by physicians at every institution to optimize the MR protocol to provide the best and most consistent quality images for that scanner/coil combination.

mpMRI Exam Protocol

A mpMRI exam combines anatomic T1 and T2 weighted imaging with functional imaging techniques such as diffusion weighted imaging (DWI) and dynamic contrast enhanced MRI (DCE-MRI). MR Spectroscopy (MRS) is no longer recommended as a part of routine prostate MRI exam under PI-RADS v2. The sequences used in mpMRI are briefly discussed below and the technical specifications for these sequences are summarized in Table 3.1.

Table 3.1 Summary of technical considerations

T2 w images
• Pulse sequence: 2D fast-spin echo or turbo-spin echo (3D sequence may be used as an adjunct)
• Imaging planes: Multiplanar axial, sagittal, coronal planes
• Field of view: 12–20 cm (to cover entire prostate and seminal vesicles)
• Slice thickness: ≤3 mm, no slice gap (location should be same as those used for DWI and DCE-MRI)
• In-plane resolution: ≤0.7 mm (phase) × ≤0.4 mm (frequency)
Diffusion weighted imaging (DWI)
• Pulse sequence: Free-breathing spin echo echo planar imaging (EPI) sequence with spectral fat saturation
• Imaging planes: Axial
• Field of view: 16–22 cm (to cover entire prostate and seminal vesicles)
• Slice thickness: ≤4 mm, no slice gap (location should be same as those used for T2w and DCE-MRI)
• Time of echo (TE): ≤90 ms; Time of repetition (TR): ≥3000 ms
• In-plane resolution: ≤2.5 mm (phase and frequency)
• b-values: At least two b-values for creating ADC map, lower b-value at 50–100 s/mm^2 and other at 800–1000 s/mm^2. Additional high b-values images (≥1400 s/mm^2) may be acquired separately or extrapolated from lower b-value (1000 s/mm^2) images
Dynamic contrast enhanced imaging (DCE-MRI)
• Pulse sequence: Either a 2D or 3D T1 weighted gradient echo (GRE) sequence may be used, 3D is preferred
• Imaging planes: Axial
• Field of view: Cover entire prostate and seminal vesicles
• Slice thickness: 3 mm, no slice gap (location should be same as those used for T2w and DCE-MRI)
• TR/TE: <100 ms/<5 ms
• In-plane resolution: ≤2 mm × ≤2 mm
• Temporal resolution: ≤15 s (<7–10 s is preferred)
• Total observation time: >2 min
• Contrast dose: 0.1 mmol/kg standard gadolinium based contrast agent
• Injection rate: 2–3 cc/s staling with continuous image data acquisition (should be the same for all exams)

Anatomic T1 Weighted and T2 Weighted Images

Axial T1 weighted image is essential to detect post-biopsy hemorrhage. T1 weighted images may be acquired with or without fat suppression and should match the locations of T2 weighted and diffusion weighted imaging (DWI). However, T1 weighted images can have lower spatial resolution compared to T2 weighted and DWI (Figs. 3.1 and 3.2).

Multiplanar T2 weighted images (axial, sagittal, coronal) are essential for evaluation of zonal anatomy, assessment of prostate gland and local staging of tumor (e.g: seminal vesicle invasion, extracapsular spread of tumor and neurovascular bundle involvement) (Fig. 3.3).

Technical Considerations Multiplanar 2D fast spin echo (FSE) images, with small field of view (12–20 cm) and 3 mm slice thickness, are recommended. Both straight axial to the patient and oblique axial images perpendicular to the long-axis of the

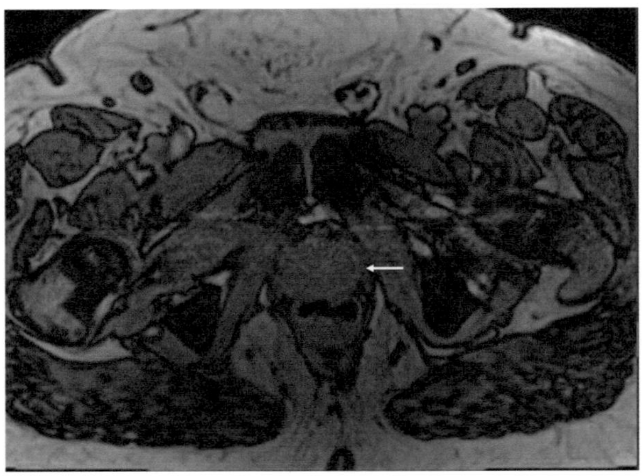

Fig. 3.1 T1 weighted gradient echo image of the prostate (arrow)

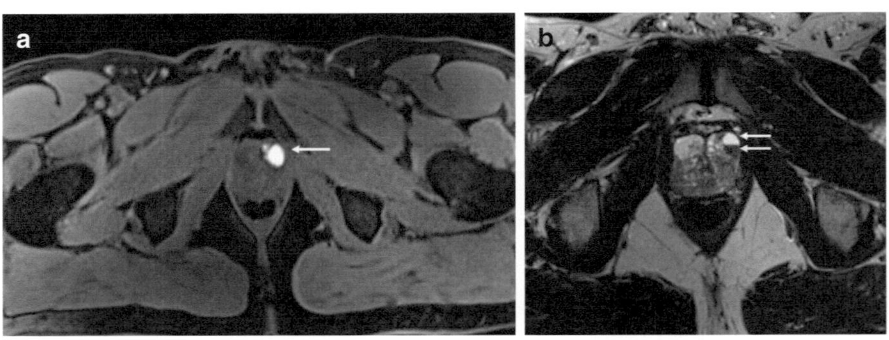

Fig. 3.2 T1 weighted fat saturated gradient echo image shows hemorrhage seen as a bright lesion in left apex of prostate (arrow, **a**). On the corresponding T2 weighted image, alternate dark and bright blood-fluid level (arrows, **b**) is seen, which is characteristic for hemorrhage

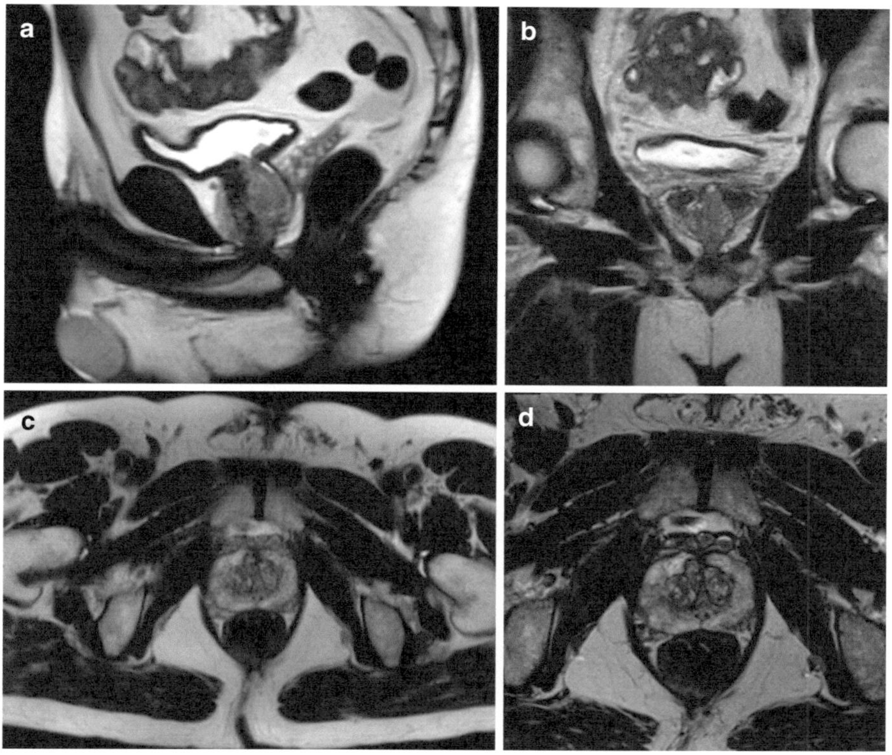

Fig. 3.3 Multiplanar T2 weighted large field of view single shot spin echo images show the prostate in sagittal (**a**), coronal (**b**) and axial (**c**) planes. Figure (**d**) shows a small field-of-view high-resolution axial section of prostate which allows better demonstration of prostate zones and internal architecture

prostate are considered acceptable. At least one additional orthogonal plane (coronal/sagittal) is recommended. The two sets of T2 weighted images (axial and coronal/sagittal) can also be used for calculating the prostate volume [4]. Volumetric 3D FSE may be used as an adjunct to multiplanar 2D FSE images and the data may be reconstructed in other planes to save overall examination time. However the reconstructed images may have a lower soft tissue contrast and lower in-plane spatial resolution as compared to 2D FSE images and thus should serve as an add-on sequence instead of replacing the high-resolution 2D T2 FSE images.

Diffusion Weighted Imaging (DWI) with Apparent Diffusion Coefficient (ADC) Maps

Diffusion is the net movement of substance from a region of higher concentration to a region lower concentration. Diffusion weighted imaging is sensitized to the movement of water molecules by using diffusion-encoding gradients of increasing strengths and/or increased duration, the combined effect of which leads to motion-related signal decay on MR images. The degree of sensitivity or weighting in an image due to diffusion is described by a "b-value" (s/mm^2), which is a calculated parameter that depends on certain user-defined settings utilized to obtain the diffusion sensitivity. The signal loss due to diffusion is greater when higher b-values are used and when the substance or tissue has a higher diffusivity. Diffusion weighted images at different b-values can be used to calculate the apparent diffusion coefficient. The diffusivity measured by MR is termed the "apparent" diffusivity because any movement of molecules, even if non-diffusive, can contribute to the signal loss that is used to calculate the coefficient.

Normal prostate tissue is rich in glandular lumen space, which allows relatively unhindered diffusion of water molecules within these spaces, and thus apparent diffusion coefficient in normal prostate is relatively high compared to many tissues. Qualitatively, normal prostate looks dark on high b-value image and bright on corresponding apparent diffusion coefficient map (Fig. 3.4). On the other hand,

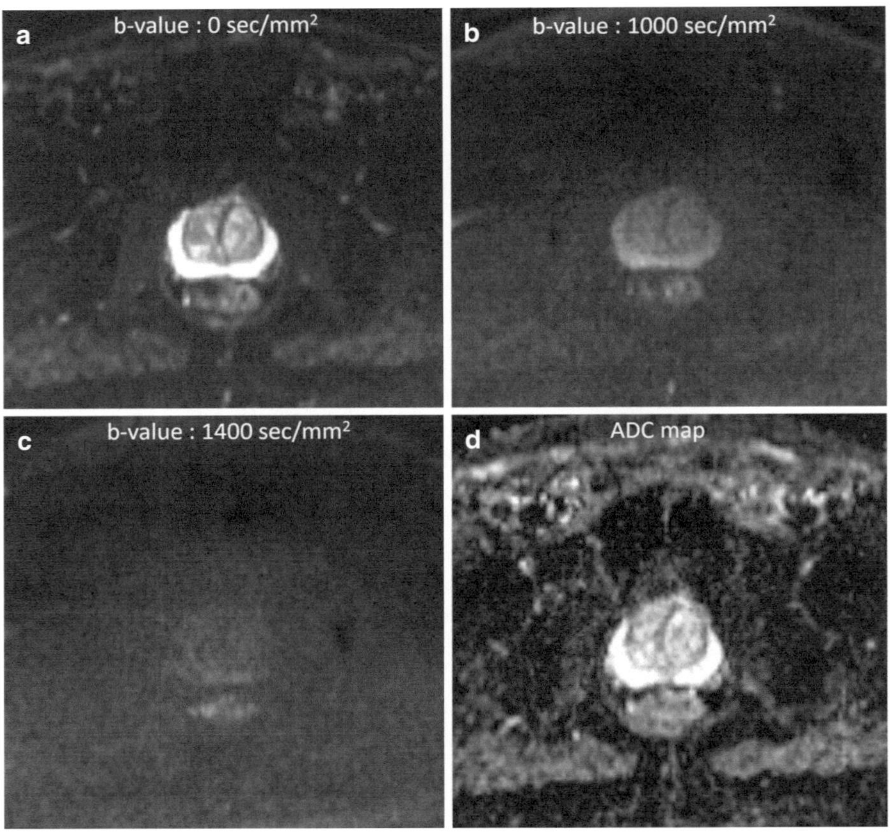

Fig. 3.4 Diffusion weighted images acquired at b-values 50, 1000 and 1400 s/mm^2 (**a–c**) with the corresponding apparent diffusion coefficient (ADC) map (**d**). At high b-values the background normal prostate signal is suppressed which allows cancer to be seen as bright lesions

in prostate cancer, tissue cellularity increases which impedes the motion of water, and there is a decrease in the apparent diffusion coefficient as compared to normal prostate. Thus cancerous tissue appears bright on high b-value images and dark on the apparent diffusion coefficient map [11, 12].

Apparent diffusion coefficient maps also provide quantitative information and various studies have shown inverse correlation between apparent diffusion coefficient values and higher Gleason grades of prostate cancer [13–19]. Apparent diffusion coefficient values have also been used to differentiate between prostatitis and prostate cancer [20–22]. However, due to overlap in apparent diffusion coefficient values between cancer and inflammation and differences in tissue composition of peripheral zone and transition zone, it is not possible to have an absolute single-value threshold for differentiation [20, 23]. Apparent diffusion coefficient values also depend on the range of b-values used, magnetic field strength and type of coil used. Thus apparent diffusion coefficient values may not be universally reproducible across various vendors. PI-RADS v2 recommends developing tailored diffusion weighted imaging protocols specific to each scanner at every institution and consistent windowing of apparent diffusion coefficient maps such that clinically significant cancers look dark or "black" on apparent diffusion coefficient maps (Fig. 3.5). *While PI-RADS v2 lays more emphasis on visual assessment of apparent diffusion coefficient maps, it also recommends that apparent diffusion coefficient threshold of 750–900 x* $10^{-6} mm^2/s$ *may be used to differentiate clinically significant cancers from prostatitis in the peripheral zone*. For evaluation of transition zone cancers, diffusion weighted imaging is given secondary importance to T2 weighted images, due to overlap in apparent diffusion coefficient values and diffusion weighted imaging appearances between benign stromal hyperplastic nodules and transition zone cancers.

The advantages of diffusion-weighted imaging are that it is simple to implement and interpret, universally available on modern MR scanners and has high image

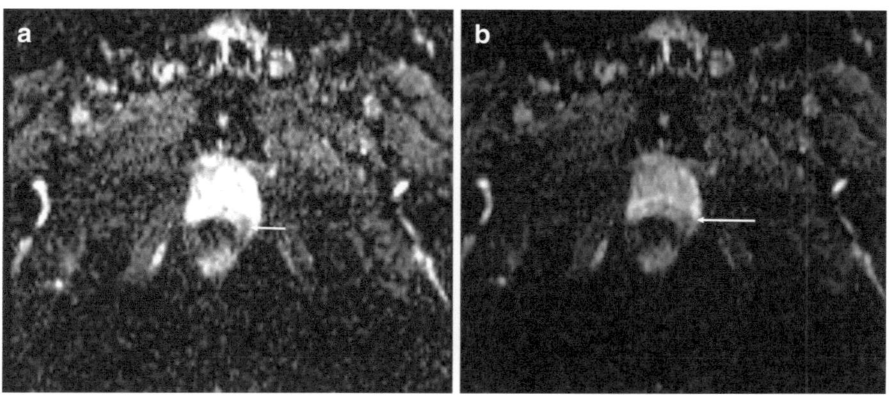

Fig. 3.5 The importance of appropriate windowing of apparent diffusion coefficient maps. Figure (**a**) shows that the apparent diffusion coefficient map output from the scanner is too bright which limits visualization of a focal suspicious lesion in left midgland region (arrow). However after appropriate windowing (**b**), the focal dark lesion is better visualized (arrow, **b**). This lesion was biopsied and turned out o be Gleason 3 + 4 = 7 prostate cancer

contrast between clinically significant prostate cancer and normal prostate tissue. However, diffusion weighted imaging is also prone to susceptibility artifacts due to gas in the rectum, presence of the endorectal coil and metallic hip implants, which can cause image distortion and artifacts (Fig. 3.6). Inadequate suppression of background signal of prostate can also affect visualization of focal lesions (Fig. 3.7). Diffusion weighted imaging is also very sensitive to motion artifacts, which can be minimized by using faster imaging techniques (single shot echo planar imaging and parallel imaging techniques). Finally, benign changes such as calcification, fibrosis, atrophy, post-biopsy hemorrhage and inflammation can also have low apparent diffusion coefficient values and may be mistaken for cancers. However, in contrast to cancers, these also appear dark on high b-value images [24].

Technical Considerations As noted above, diffusion weighted imaging is performed using a single-shot echoplanar imaging (EPI) technique. It is recommended to have

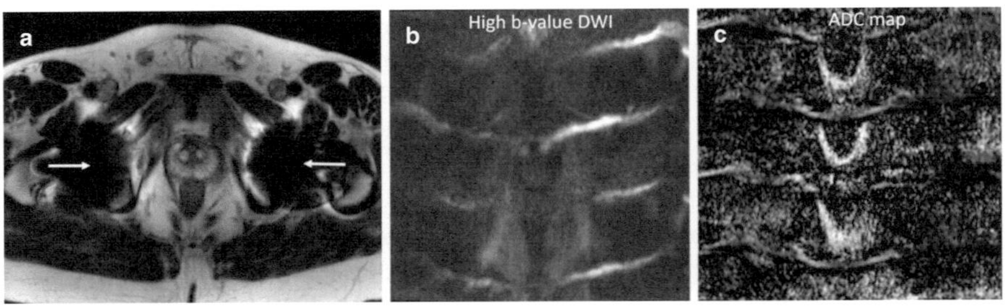

Fig. 3.6 MRI of patient with bilateral hip implants (arrows, **a**). The implants are seen as susceptibility artifacts on T2 weighted turbo spin echo (**a**) images and cause complete distortion of diffusion weighted images (**b**) and apparent diffusion coefficient (ADC) map (**c**)

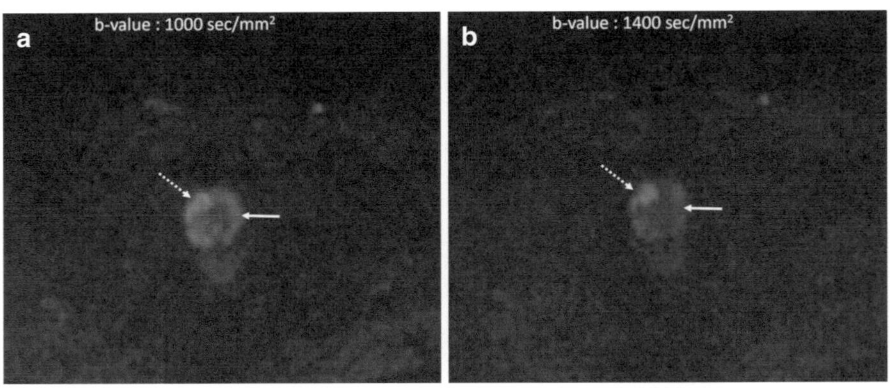

Fig. 3.7 Importance of adequate background suppression for depiction of focal lesions. Diffusion weighted image obtained at b-value of 1000 s/mm^2 (**a**) shows inadequate suppression of background prostate signal and poor visualization of focal lesion seen in right anterior apical prostate (dotted arrow). However at higher b-value of 1400 s/mm^2, the lesion is much better visualized (dotted arrow) with complete suppression of background signal (arrow, **b**)

slice thicknesses and locations comparable to T2 weighted images for easier interpretation. PI-RADSv2 recommends obtaining at least two b-value images to calculate the apparent diffusion coefficient, the lower b-value being set at at 0–100 s/mm^2 (preferably 50–100 s/mm^2) and the higher b-value at 800–1000 s/mm^2. In addition, it is also recommended to obtain ultra-high b-value images (b values at 1400–2000 s/mm^2) as this increases conspicuity of clinically significant cancers, more so in the transition zone [25–27] (Fig. 3.8). The ultra-high b-value may be acquired separately so as not to impair the appearance of apparent diffusion coefficient map obtained with the lower b-values dataset, or it may be extrapolated or calculated by the computer from the diffusion weighted imaging dataset obtained with lower b-values.

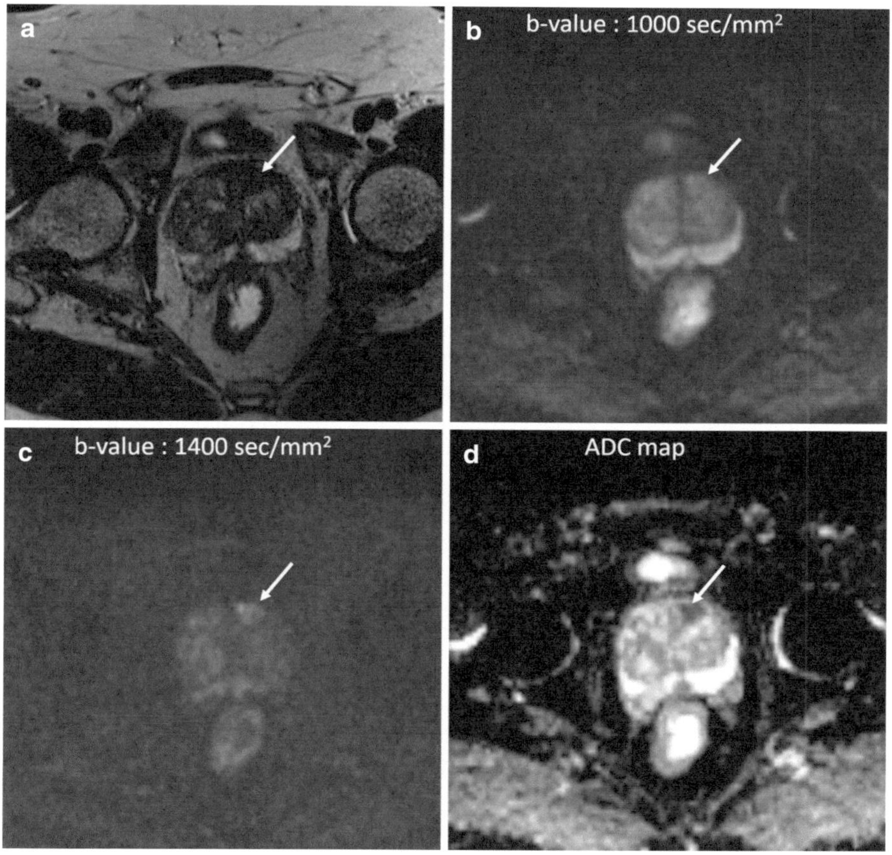

Fig. 3.8 Utility of ultra-high b-value in detection of transition zone cancers. Axial T2 weighted turbo spin echo image (**a**) shows a focal dark lesion in left anterior transition zone, which is not well seen on diffusion weighted image at b-value of 1000 s/mm^2. The lesion shows conspicuous bright signal at ultra-high b-value of 1400 s/mm^2 and is dark on corresponding apparent diffusion coefficient (ADC) map. The combination of signal intensity on T2 weighted image (**a**) and diffusion weighted images makes this lesion highly suspicious for cancer and was proven to be Gleason score 7 (3 + 4 = 7) prostate cancer on biopsy

Dynamic Contrast Enhanced (DCE)-MRI

DCE-MRI assesses vascularity and perfusion by measuring contrast kinetics before and after administration of gadolinium-based contrast agent (GBCA). Cancer is associated with neo-angiogenesis, which is depicted as early contrast enhancement compared to normal tissue. DCE-MRI comprises of a series of 3D volumetric T1 weighted images, which are acquired rapidly before and after administration of contrast. In contrast to PI-RADS v2 that recommended a high temporal resolution (7–10 s/volume), PI-RADS v2.1 considers a temporal resolution of $\leq$15 s/volume as an acceptable trade-off between adequate spatial and temporal resolution [4]. At least 2 min of continuous scanning is recommended to capture contrast dynamics soon after injection. DCE-MR images are viewed on software that allows evaluation of each slice through all time points, and identification of foci of early enhancement. It is also recommended to use fat suppression or subtraction of contrast from pre-contrast images to improve visualization of small, early enhancing lesions. Since hemorrhage can also be bright on pre-contrast T1 weighted images, and can obscure contrast enhancement, subtraction techniques can eliminate the confounding effects of hemorrhage (Fig. 3.9).

PI-RADS v2 moves away from semi-quantitative or quantitative analysis of DCE-MRI because these methods have not proven to add value to image interpretation. Moreover, quantitative analysis requires standardized acquisition techniques and sophisticated software for analysis, which may not be available everywhere. Hence under PI-RADS v2, DCE-MRI is analyzed visually. A "positive" DCE-MRI lesion shows enhancement which is focal and earlier or contemporary with adjacent prostate tissue. It must also correspond to a lesion on T2 weighted and/or diffusion weighted images. Thus under PI-RADS v2, DCE-MRI has secondary importance to T2 weighted images and diffusion weighted images and is never interpreted in isolation. DCE-MRI becomes more important when diffusion weighted images are distorted and of suboptimal quality (Fig. 3.10). A "negative" DCE-MRI lesion is one, which does not show early enhancement or shows diffuse enhancement not corresponding to any focal abnormality on T2 weighted and/or diffusion weighted imaging.

Technical Considerations DCE-MRI is acquired using a T1 weighted gradient echo sequence, since these can be rapidly acquired. While both 2D and 3D sequences may be used, 3D is preferred for volumetric coverage. The craniocaudal coverage should be same as T2 weighted and diffusion weighted images, but DCE-MRI can have a lower in-plane resolution. While PI-RADSv2 recommends a high temporal resolution, with whole prostate being scanned rapidly and repeatedly every 7–10 s with at least 2 min of continuous scanning, PI-RADS v2.1 considers a temporal resolution < 15 s as adequate. In practice, faster scan times are preferred for better assessment of enhancement timings. Either fat suppression or subtraction technique is recommended to improve lesion conspicuity.

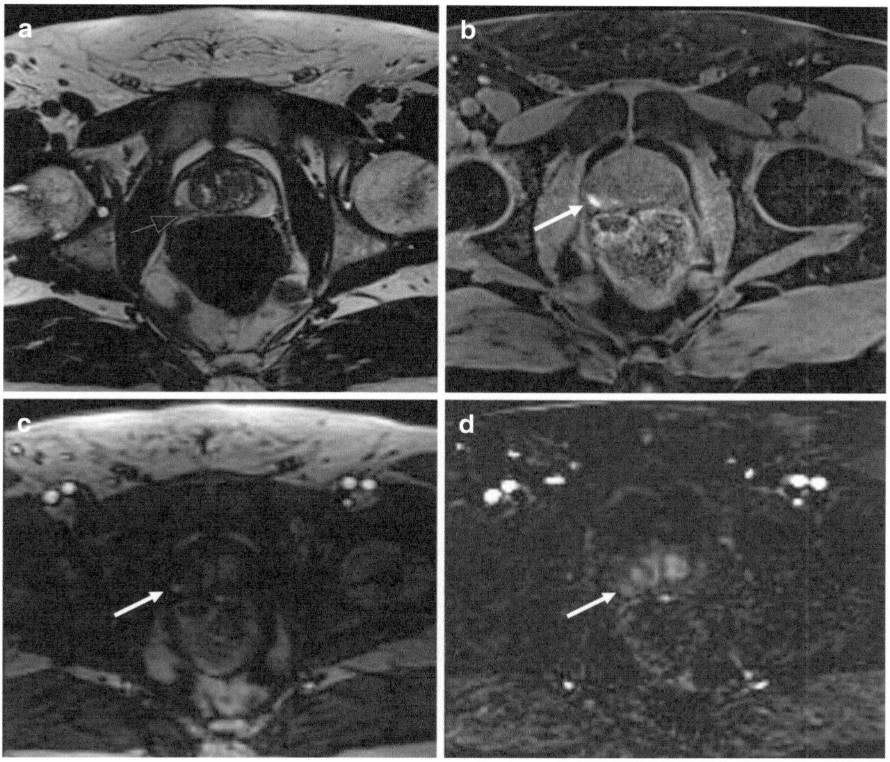

Fig. 3.9 Utility of subtracted dynamic contrast enhanced images. Axial T2 weighted turbo spin echo image (**a**) shows a focal dark abnormality in right peripheral zone (arrow, **a**). On T1 weighted image, there is hemorrhage at that location (arrow, **b**). Presence of hemorrhage confounds interpretation of post-contrast dynamic contrast enhanced (DCE) image (**c**) as the bright signal can either represent hemorrhage or contrast enhancement. However subtracted DCE image (**d**) confirms there is contrast enhancement in that location, suggestive of cancer. Biopsy showed prostate cancer with Gleason score 3 + 3 = 6

Diagnostic Accuracy of mpMRI of Prostate

Even before the PI-RADS committee devised the structured scoring system for evaluating mpMRI, various studies explored the role of mpMRI for detection, localization and staging of prostate cancer. These studies evaluated the diagnostic performance of a T2 weighted sequence alone, followed by a combination of T2 weighted + diffusion weighted imaging and/or T2 weighted + DCE-MRI or all three sequences together in detecting/localizing prostate cancer, using radical prostatectomy or biopsies as gold standard for comparison. Overall most authors found that that a combination of T2 weighted and diffusion weighted imaging had improved diagnostic performance compared to T2 weighted imaging alone [28–30]. Using a

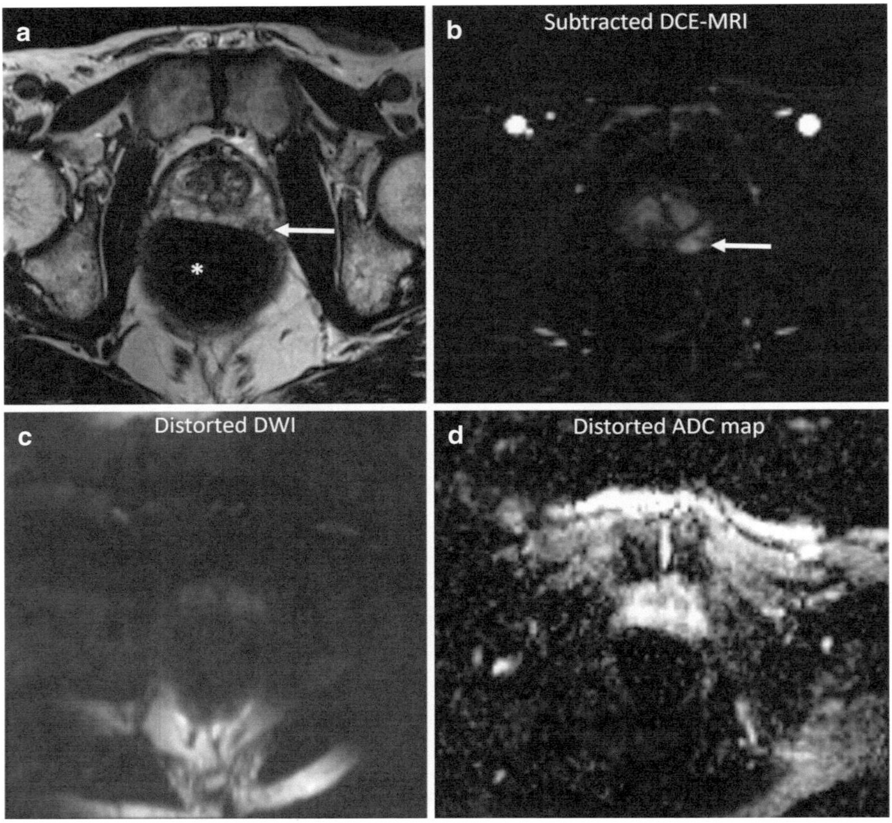

Fig. 3.10 Utility of dynamic contrast enhanced (DCE)- MRI when diffusion weighted imaging is not interpretable. Axial T2 weighted image (**a**) shows a focal dark lesion in left peripheral zone (arrow) which shows enhancement on subtracted DCE-MRI (**b**). Due to gas in rectum (asterisk, **a**), the diffusion weighted image (**c**) and apparent diffusion coefficient (ADC) map (**d**) are distorted and cannot be interpreted. In such a scenario, the combination of focal lesion on T2 weighted image with early enhancement in peripheral zone is highly suspicious for malignancy and needs to be biopsied. This was a biopsy proven Gleason 6 (3 + 3 = 6) prostate cancer

combination of T2 weighted and diffusion weighted imaging was found to be more helpful in the peripheral zone as compared to transition zone [28, 29]. In a recent meta-analysis on the accuracy of mpMRI for prostate cancer detection, mpMRI was found to have a pooled specificity of 0.88 (95% CI, 0.82–0.92) and sensitivity of 0.74 (95% CI, 0.66–0.81) for prostate cancer detection, with negative predictive values ranging from 0.65 to 0.94 [31]. In summary, adding diffusion weighted imaging has been shown to increase sensitivity as well as specificity for detection and localization of clinically significant cancers while DCE-MRI may improve diagnostic accuracy by detecting smaller or more aggressive cancers [32, 33].

References

1. Barentsz JO, Richenberg J, Clements R, Choyke P, Verma S, Villeirs G, et al. ESUR prostate MR guidelines 2012. Eur Radiol. 2012;22(4):746–57.
2. Barrett T, Turkbey B, Choyke PL. PI-RADS version 2: what you need to know. Clin Radiol. 2015;70(11):1165–76.
3. ACR, ESUR, AdMeTech Foundation. Prostate imaging and reporting and data system: version 2. 2014. Available at 12/9/2016, http://www.acr.org/w/media/ACR/Documents/PDF/QualitySafety/Resources/PIRADS/PIRADS%20V2.pdf [Internet]. [cited 2016 Dec 9]. Available at 14/4/2015, http://www.acr.org/w/media/ACR/Documents/PDF/QualitySafety/Resources/PIRADS/PIRADS%20V2.pdf.
4. Turkbey B, Rosenkrantz AB, Haider MA, Padhani AR, Villeirs G, Macura KJ, et al. Prostate imaging reporting and data system version 2.1: 2019 update of prostate imaging reporting and data system version 2. Eur Urol [Internet]. 2019 Mar 18 [cited 2019 Jun 27]. https://www.europeanurology.com/article/S0302-2838(19)30180-0/abstract.
5. Tamada T, Sone T, Jo Y, Yamamoto A, Yamashita T, Egashira N, et al. Prostate cancer: relationships between postbiopsy hemorrhage and tumor detectability at MR diagnosis. Radiology. 2008;248(2):531–9.
6. Qayyum A, Coakley FV, Lu Y, Olpin JD, Wu L, Yeh BM, et al. Organ-confined prostate cancer: effect of prior transrectal biopsy on endorectal MRI and MR spectroscopic imaging. AJR Am J Roentgenol. 2004;183(4):1079–83.
7. Ikonen S, Kivisaari L, Vehmas T, Tervahartiala P, Salo JO, Taari K, et al. Optimal timing of post-biopsy MR imaging of the prostate. Acta Radiol. 2001;42(1):70–3.
8. Barrett T, Vargas HA, Akin O, Goldman DA, Hricak H. Value of the hemorrhage exclusion sign on T1-weighted prostate MR images for the detection of prostate cancer. Radiology. 2012;263(3):751–7.
9. Rouvière O, Hartman RP, Lyonnet D. Prostate MR imaging at high-field strength: evolution or revolution? Eur Radiol. 2006;16(2):276–84.
10. Shah ZK, Elias SN, Abaza R, Zynger DL, DeRenne LA, Knopp MV, et al. Performance comparison of 1.5-T endorectal coil MRI with 3.0-T nonendorectal coil MRI in patients with prostate cancer. Acad Radiol. 2015;22(4):467–74.
11. Gibbs P, Tozer DJ, Liney GP, Turnbull LW. Comparison of quantitative T2 mapping and diffusion-weighted imaging in the normal and pathologic prostate. Magn Reson Med. 2001;46(6):1054–8.
12. Zelhof B, Pickles M, Liney G, Gibbs P, Rodrigues G, Kraus S, et al. Correlation of diffusion-weighted magnetic resonance data with cellularity in prostate cancer. BJU Int. 2009;103(7):883–8.
13. deSouza NM, Riches SF, Vanas NJ, Morgan VA, Ashley SA, Fisher C, et al. Diffusion-weighted magnetic resonance imaging: a potential non-invasive marker of tumour aggressiveness in localized prostate cancer. Clin Radiol. 2008;63(7):774–82.
14. Bittencourt LK, Barentsz JO, de Miranda LC, Gasparetto EL. Prostate MRI: diffusion-weighted imaging at 1.5T correlates better with prostatectomy Gleason grades than TRUS-guided biopsies in peripheral zone tumours. Eur Radiol. 2012;22(2):468–75.
15. Itou Y, Nakanishi K, Narumi Y, Nishizawa Y, Tsukuma H. Clinical utility of apparent diffusion coefficient (ADC) values in patients with prostate cancer: can ADC values contribute to assess the aggressiveness of prostate cancer? J Magn Reson Imaging. 2011;33(1):167–72.
16. Verma S, Rajesh A, Morales H, Lemen L, Bills G, Delworth M, et al. Assessment of aggressiveness of prostate cancer: correlation of apparent diffusion coefficient with histologic grade after radical prostatectomy. AJR Am J Roentgenol. 2011;196(2):374–81.
17. Hambrock T, Somford DM, Huisman HJ, van Oort IM, Witjes JA, Hulsbergen-van de Kaa CA, et al. Relationship between apparent diffusion coefficients at 3.0-T MR imaging and Gleason grade in peripheral zone prostate cancer. Radiology. 2011;259(2):453–61.

18. Miao H, Fukatsu H, Ishigaki T. Prostate cancer detection with 3-T MRI: comparison of diffusion-weighted and T2-weighted imaging. Eur J Radiol. 2007;61(2):297–302.
19. Turkbey B, Shah VP, Pang Y, Bernardo M, Xu S, Kruecker J, et al. Is apparent diffusion coefficient associated with clinical risk scores for prostate cancers that are visible on 3-T MR images? Radiology. 2011;258(2):488–95.
20. Nagel KNA, Schouten MG, Hambrock T, Litjens GJS, Hoeks CMA, ten Haken B, et al. Differentiation of prostatitis and prostate cancer by using diffusion-weighted MR imaging and MR-guided biopsy at 3 T. Radiology. 2013;267(1):164–72.
21. Kim CK, Park BK, Han JJ, Kang TW, Lee HM. Diffusion-weighted imaging of the prostate at 3 T for Differentiation of malignant and benign tissue in transition and peripheral zones: preliminary results. J Comput Assist Tomogr. 2007;31(3):449–54.
22. Esen M, Onur MR, Akpolat N, Orhan I, Kocakoc E. Utility of ADC measurement on diffusion-weighted MRI in differentiation of prostate cancer, normal prostate and prostatitis. Quant Imaging Med Surg. 2013;3(4):210–6.
23. Hoeks CMA, Vos EK, Bomers JGR, Barentsz JO, Hulsbergen-van de Kaa CA, Scheenen TW. Diffusion-weighted magnetic resonance imaging in the prostate transition zone: histopathological validation using magnetic resonance–guided biopsy specimens. Investig Radiol. 2013;48(10):693–701.
24. Kitzing YX, Prando A, Varol C, Karczmar GS, Maclean F, Oto A. Benign conditions that mimic prostate carcinoma: MR imaging features with histopathologic correlation. Radiographics. 2015;36(1):162–75.
25. Koo JH, Kim CK, Choi D, Park BK, Kwon GY, Kim B. Diffusion-weighted magnetic resonance imaging for the evaluation of prostate cancer: optimal B value at 3T. Korean J Radiol. 2013;14(1):61–9.
26. Metens T, Miranda D, Absil J, Matos C. What is the optimal b value in diffusion-weighted MR imaging to depict prostate cancer at 3T? Eur Radiol. 2012;22(3):703–9.
27. Ueno Y, Kitajima K, Sugimura K, Kawakami F, Miyake H, Obara M, et al. Ultra-high b-value diffusion-weighted MRI for the detection of prostate cancer with 3-T MRI. J Magn Reson Imaging. 2013;38(1):154–60.
28. Haider MA, van der Kwast TH, Tanguay J, Evans AJ, Hashmi A-T, Lockwood G, et al. Combined T2-weighted and diffusion-weighted MRI for localization of prostate cancer. Am J Roentgenol. 2007;189(2):323–8.
29. Delongchamps NB, Rouanne M, Flam T, Beuvon F, Liberatore M, Zerbib M, et al. Multiparametric magnetic resonance imaging for the detection and localization of prostate cancer: combination of T2-weighted, dynamic contrast-enhanced and diffusion-weighted imaging. BJU Int. 2011;107(9):1411–8.
30. Lim HK, Kim JK, Kim KA, Cho K-S. Prostate cancer: apparent diffusion coefficient map with T2-weighted images for detection--a multireader study. Radiology. 2009;250(1):145–51.
31. de Rooij M, Hamoen EHJ, Witjes JA, Barentsz JO, Rovers MM. Accuracy of magnetic resonance imaging for local staging of prostate cancer: a diagnostic meta-analysis. Eur Urol. 2016;70(2):233–45.
32. Hötker AM, Mazaheri Y, Aras Ö, Zheng J, Moskowitz CS, Gondo T, et al. Assessment of prostate cancer aggressiveness by use of the combination of quantitative DWI and dynamic contrast-enhanced MRI. AJR Am J Roentgenol. 2016;206(4):756–63.
33. Kitajima K, Kaji Y, Fukabori Y, Yoshida K, Suganuma N, Sugimura K. Prostate cancer detection with 3 T MRI: comparison of diffusion-weighted imaging and dynamic contrast-enhanced MRI in combination with T2-weighted imaging. J Magn Reson Imaging. 2010;31(3):625–31.

4 Multiparametric MRI of Prostate: Analysis and Recommendations of Prostate Imaging Reporting and Data System (PI-RADS) Version 2.1

Ananya Panda and Vikas Gulani

Multiparametric MRI, comprising of anatomic T1 weighted and T2 weighted imaging combined with functional imaging techniques, presently diffusion weighted imaging and dynamic contrast enhanced (DCE) MRI, is the standard of care for evaluation of prostate cancer. Efforts have been taken to standardize prostate MRI reporting and interpretation by the international community comprising of both radiologists and urologists. These efforts have led to consensus guidelines in the shape of PI-RADS recommendations, the second version of which was released in 2015. PI-RADS v2 recommendations and subsequent PI-RADS v2.1 updates are geared towards detection of *clinically significant cancer*. Clinically significant cancer is defined as cancer with Gleason score $\geq 3 + 4 = 7$, tumor volume >0.5 ml, and/or extraprostatic extension. PI-RADS v2.1 defines primary and secondary MR sequences for both peripheral zone and transition zone, enumerates findings on these sequences that are definitely benign or have increasing probability of cancer and recommends an overall 1–5 scoring system where a score 1 indicates a very low probability and score 5 indicates a very high probability of clinically significant cancer.

In this chapter, the assessment of peripheral zone and transition zone, using various MR sequences, and MR staging and reporting of prostate cancer are described in detail.

A. Panda
Department of Radiology, Mayo Clinic, Rochester, MN, USA
e-mail: panda.ananya@mayo.edu

V. Gulani (✉)
Fred Jenner Hodges Professor and Chair, Department of Radiology, University of Michigan, Ann Arbor, MI, USA
e-mail: vikasgulani@med.umich.edu

A. Panda et al. (eds.), *Reading MRI of the Prostate*,
https://doi.org/10.1007/978-3-319-99357-7_4

Sequence Assessment

T2 Weighted Images

Peripheral Zone Normal peripheral zone has a high signal intensity on T2 weighted images whereas prostate cancers have low signal intensity due to decreased water content. To correctly identify peripheral zone prostate cancers, PI-RADS v2 recommends looking at shape, borders and extent of lesions on T2 weighted imaging [1] (Table 4.1, Fig. 4.1).

Prostate cancers in the peripheral zone appear as focal, round or lenticular, mass-like, circumscribed lesions with homogeneously and moderately decreased signal intensity. In general, more aggressive cancers are more conspicuous and distinctly seen on T2 weighted images. In addition, lesion size has been positively correlated with Gleason grade and extraprostatic extension [2, 3]. Hence PI-RADS v2 uses a size cut-off of 1.5 cm to upgrade overall PI-RADS score from 4 to 5. In addition, any lesion with extracapsular extension or seminal vesicle invasion is automatically scored 5 irrespective of lesion size.

Benign pathologies such as prostatitis often appear as linear, wedge-shaped, or diffuse lesions with mildly low signal intensity and indistinct borders (Fig. 4.2). Similarly, post-biopsy hemorrhage can also appear indistinctly dark on T2 weighted images. More importantly, hemorrhage appears bright on corresponding T1 weighted images. In addition, cancers often demonstrate a "halo" sign or "hemorrhage exclusion" on T1 weighted images wherein cancers appear as a focal, well-defined isointense mass surrounded by a halo of hyperintense hemorrhage [4].

Despite these differences between cancer and benign conditions on high resolution T2 weighted images, overlap in appearance does exist between cancerous and non-cancerous lesions. Thus a T2 weighted sequence alone has only moderate

Table 4.1 T2 weighted scoring for peripheral zone lesions

Score	Shape	Signal intensity	Size/extra-prostatic extension	Figures
1	N/A	High Homogeneous	N/A	Fig. 4.1a
2	Linear/ wedge-shaped Diffuse Indistinct	Mild-moderate low Heterogeneous	Any size No extraprostatic extension	Fig. 4.1b, c
3	Round Non-circumscribed Diffuse	Moderate low Heterogeneous	Any size No extraprostatic extension	Fig. 4.1d
4	Focus/mass Circumscribed	Moderate low Homogeneous	Size <1.5 cm in greatest dimension	Fig. 4.1e
5	Focus/mass Circumscribed	Moderate low Homogeneous	Size ≥1.5 cm in greatest dimension and/or extraprostatic extension present	Fig. 4.1f

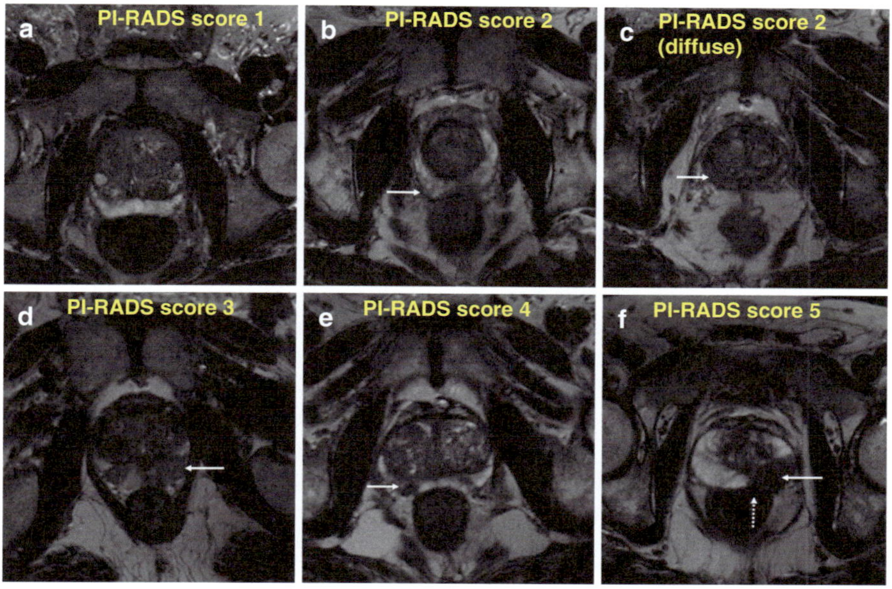

Fig. 4.1 T2 weighted scoring system for peripheral zone. Axial T2 weighted images (**a**–**f**) show examples of PI-RADS 1 (**a**), PI-RADS 2 (**b**, **c**), PI-RADS 3 (**d**), PI-RADS 4 (**e**) and PI-RADS 5 lesion (**f**) with extracapsular extension (dotted arrow, **f**) in the peripheral zone of the prostate. PI-RADS 3 on T2 weighted image refers to diffuse or wedge-shaped lobar lesion with moderate dark signal. PI-RADS 4 and 5 lesions refer to focal lesions with very dark appearance less than (**e**) or greater than 1.5 cm respectively (**f**)

Fig. 4.2 Axial T2 weighted image shows sharply defined, wedge-shaped lesions in left peripheral zone (arrows) which are characteristic for prostatitis and are scored as PI-RADS 2 and do not require biopsy

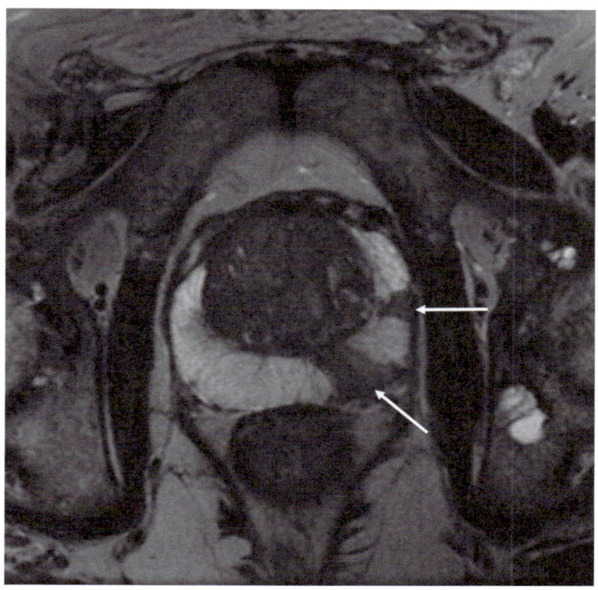

diagnostic accuracy for cancer detection and diagnostic performance is significantly improved when T2 weighted imaging is combined with diffusion weighted imaging and/or DCE-MRI [5–8].

The T2 weighted scoring system for peripheral zone lesions and the corresponding MR examples have been depicted in Table 4.1 and Fig. 4.1a–f.

Transition Zone Transition zone cancers are less common than peripheral zone, but still comprise 25–30% of all prostate cancers. Evaluation of transition zone cancers on anatomic T2 weighted sequences is complicated by the fact that the transition zone also undergoes benign prostatic hyperplasia (BPH). The hyperplastic nodules cause the transition zone to have a very heterogeneous and bizarre appearance on T2 weighted images, sometimes termed as "organized chaos" (Fig. 4.3). BPH can affect both glandular and stromal tissue and appear as band-like areas and/or encapsulated round nodules with circumscribed margins. Predominantly glandular hyperplasia has a heterogeneous appearance on T2 weighted images, with pockets of high T2 weighted signal mixed with foci of low signal (Fig. 4.4b). Stromal nodules have low signal intensity on T2 weighted imaging, and can look very similar to interspersed foci of prostate cancer (Fig. 4.4c). However, in general, most BPH nodules have an admixture of signal intensities and are sharply circumscribed and encapsulated as compared to cancer.

Under PI-RADS 2.1 update, the typical looking BPH nodules are scored as Category 1 lesions, i.e. clinical cancer is highly unlikely (Table 4.2). Focal lesions in the transition zone are only scored if they have morphology known to be associated with

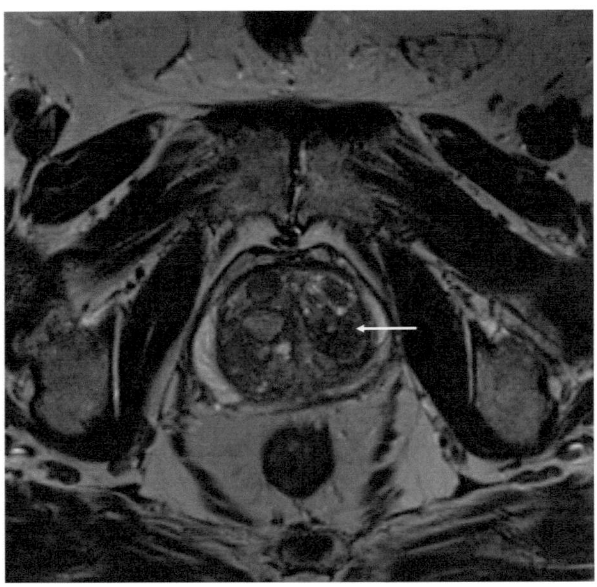

Fig. 4.3 Axial T2 weighted image shows hypertrophied transition zone with multiple well-defined capsulated nodules and very heterogeneous signal intensity with bright and dark areas corresponding to the "organized chaos" description for benign prostatic hypertrophy. This appearance is scored PI-RADS 1 and is a normal finding

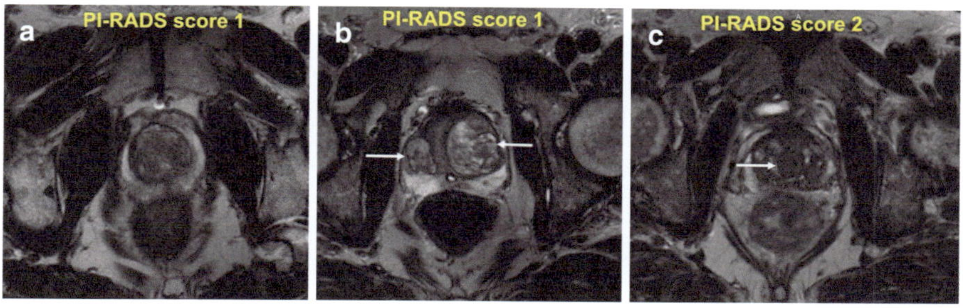

Fig. 4.4 PI-RADS 1 and 2 scores for transition zone on T2 weighted images. PI-RADS 1 (**a**) refers to transition zone with homogeneous appearance and intermediate signal intensity and to circumscribed nodule that is completely encapsulated (**b**). PI-RADS 2 refers to circumscribed nodules that are either incompletely encapsulated or non-encapsulated with homogeneous low signal intensity (**c**)

Table 4.2 T2 weighted scoring for transition zone lesions

Score	Shape	Signal intensity	Size/extra-prostatic extension	Figures
1	Circumscribed completely encapsulated nodule (definite capsule seen)	Variable signal intensity, homogeneous/heterogeneous that does NOT differ from the background transition zone	N/A	Fig. 4.4a, b
2	Circumscribed nodule without encapsulation or almost encapsulated	Low/homogeneous/ heterogeneous	Any size No extra-prostatic extension	Fig. 4.4c
3	Nodule with obscured margin	Heterogeneous	Any size No extra-prostatic extension	Fig. 4.5a, b
4	Lenticular lesion Non-circumscribed margin	Moderate low Homogeneous	Size <1.5 cm in greatest dimension	Fig. 4.6a
5	Lenticular lesion Non-circumscribed margin	Moderate low Homogeneous	Size ≥ 1.5 cm in greatest dimension and/or extra-prostatic extension present	Fig. 4.6b

cancer (Table 4.2, Figs. 4.5 and 4.6) or if their appearances differ from the predominant appearance of the background transition zone on either the T2 weighted or the diffusion-weighted images [9].

Based on these findings, all circumscribed nodules with heterogeneous appearance and low/high signal intensity are scored as 1. When circumscribed nodules in the transition zone are incompletely or almost completely encapsulated, these atypical nodules are assigned a score of 2. Nodules with obscured margins and heterogeneous signal intensity are scored as 3 with equivocal risk of cancer. Non-circumscribed, ill-defined, lenticular shape lesions with irregular margins and

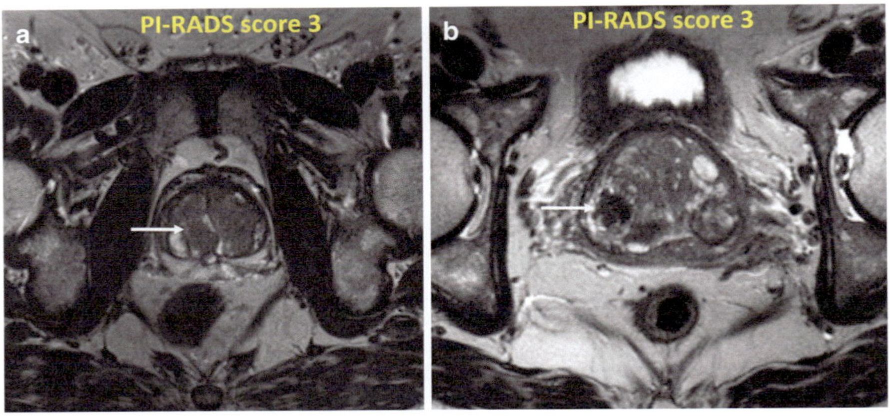

Fig. 4.5 T2 weighted score 3 for transition zone. Transition zone nodules with low signal intensity and partly obscured (**a**) or ill-defined margins (**b**) are scored as 3

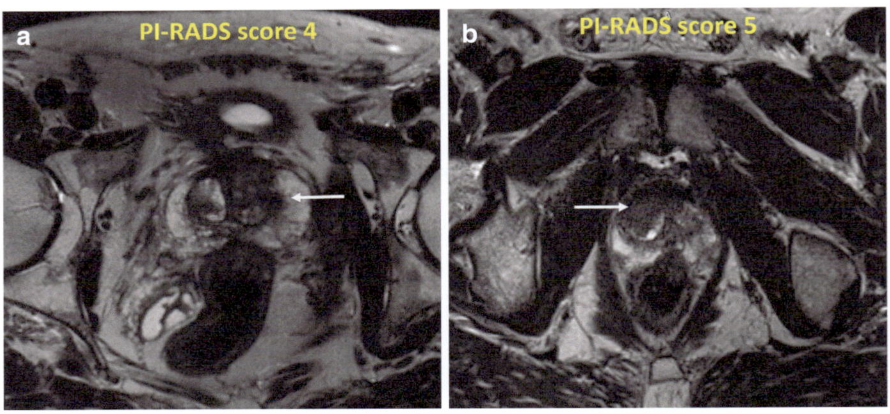

Fig. 4.6 T2 weighted score 4 and 5 for transition zone. A lenticular lesion with low signal intensity and ill-defined margins less than 1.5 cm in greatest dimension is scored as 4 (**a**) and greater than 1.5 cm is scored as 5 (**b**)

homogeneous low signal intensity are scored as 4 and above, with a size cut-off of 1.5 cm or ECE upgrading score to 5 (Table 4.2).

Diffusion Weighted Imaging with Apparent Diffusion Coefficient Map

Diffusion weighted imaging is evaluated in conjunction with an apparent diffusion coefficient map to identify lesions with restricted diffusion. PI-RADSv2 has a common scoring system for diffusion weighted imaging for both peripheral zone and transition zone lesions (Table 4.3, Fig. 4.7) and relies on subjective

Table 4.3 Diffusion weighted imaging scoring for all (peripheral and transition zone) lesions

Score	Signal intensity on high b-value diffusion weighted imaging	Signal intensity on ADC map	Size/extra-prostatic extension	Figures
1	No focal abnormality Homogeneous low	No focal abnormality Homogeneous high	N/A	Fig. 4.7a
2	Linear/wedge-shaped Mildly high	Linear/ wedge-shaped Low or indistinct	Any size No extra-prostatic extension	Fig. 4.7b
3	Focal lesion Mildly-moderately high	Focal lesion Mild-moderately low	Any size No extra-prostatic extension	Fig. 4.7c
4	Focal lesion Markedly high	Focal lesion Markedly low	Size <1.5 cm and/or extra-prostatic extension absent	Fig. 4.7d
5	Focal lesion Markedly high	Focal lesion Markedly low	Size ≥1.5 cm and/or extra-prostatic extension present	Fig. 4.7e

assessment rather than using threshold values of apparent diffusion coefficient for characterization.

Thus, a lesion is said to be diffusion restricted if it is focal, markedly bright on high b-value diffusion weighted imaging and shows markedly low apparent diffusion coefficient on diffusion mapping. Similar to T2 weighted images, a cut off of 1.5 cm or extra-prostatic extension is used to upgrade from score 4 to score 5.

Diffusion weighted imaging score 3 refers to a focal lesion which is mildly bright on diffusion weighted imaging and mildly dark on the apparent diffusion coefficient map. A lesion with score 3 may also be markedly bright on diffusion-weighted imaging OR markedly dark on apparent diffusion coefficient map but NOT both [9].

Linear/wedge shaped lesions that appear dark on apparent diffusion coefficient and/or bright on diffusion-weighted imaging are scored 2.

DCE-MRI

Despite the large number of images obtained by DCE-MRI, PI-RADS v2 underplays the role of this sequence since benign transition zone nodules and prostatitis have enhancement characteristics that can mimic cancer [10]. Currently, DCE-MRI is scored as positive/negative instead of a 5-point scoring system. DCE-MRI is viewed by scrolling through a stack of images of the prostate and following the enhancement patterns over time. Any focal lesion with early or contemporaneous enhancement to rest of prostatic tissue and correlated with focal abnormality on T2 weighted sequence and/or diffusion weighted imaging is

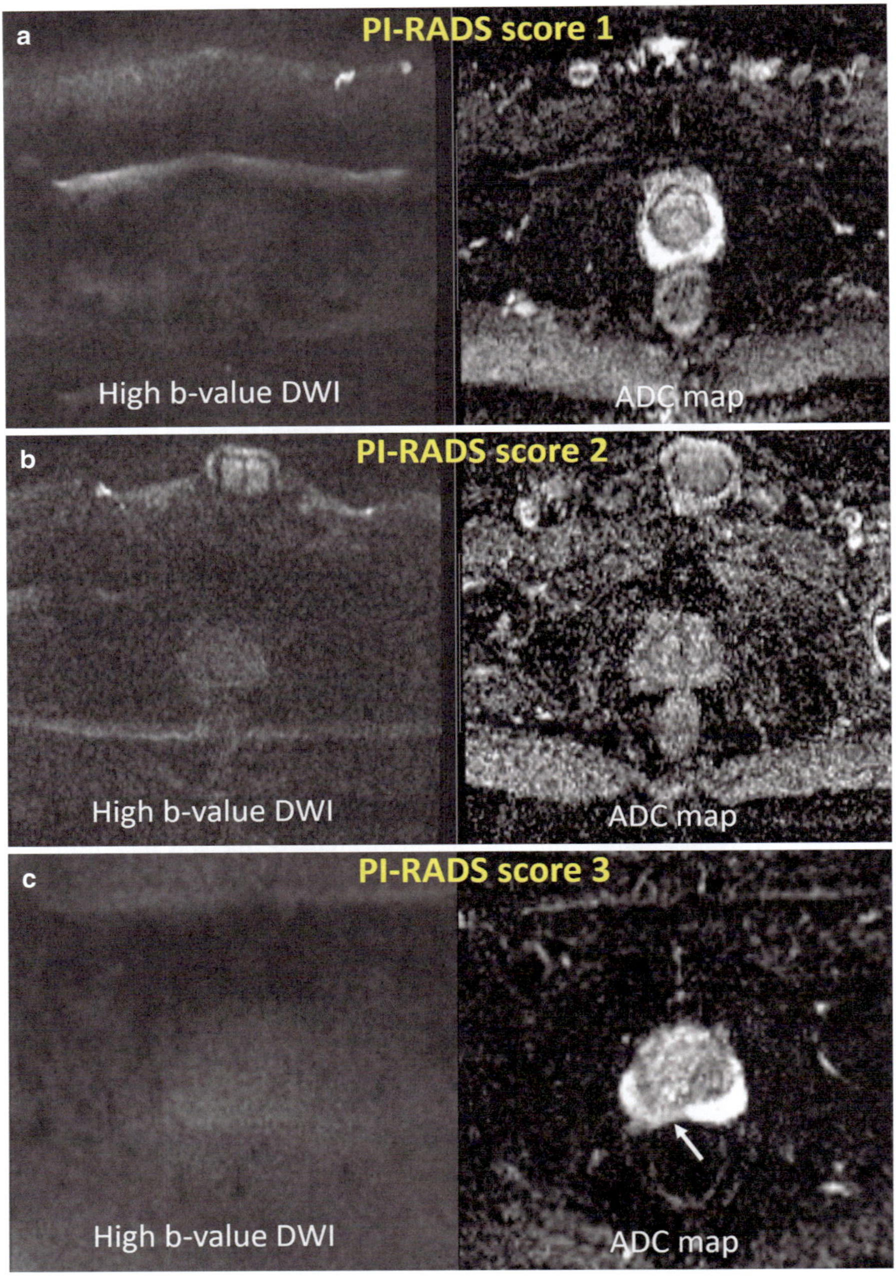

Fig. 4.7 Examples of score 1–5 lesions on high b-value diffusion weighted images (DWI) and corresponding apparent diffusion coefficient (ADC) maps. PI-RADS 1 (**a**) and PI-RADS 2 (**b**) do not show distinct abnormality on DWI or ADC maps. PI-RADS 3 on DWI refers to focal lesion which is isointense or has a mildly increased signal intensity (**c** left column) on high b-value DWI and mildly low signal intensity on ADC map (**c** right column). PI-RADS 4 and 5 scores refer to focal lesions with markedly high signal intensity on high b-value DWI and markedly low signal intensity on ADC map, less than 1.5 cm (**d**) and more than 1.5 cm (**e**) respectively

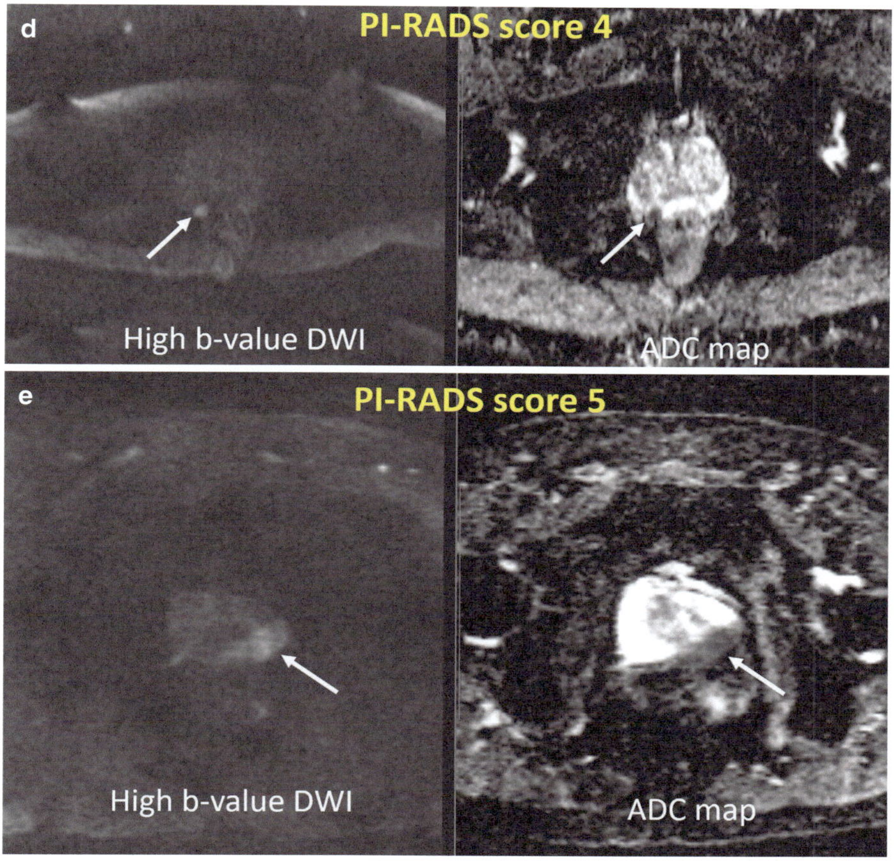

Fig. 4.7 (continued)

scored as DCE-MRI positive. For peripheral zone, DCE-MRI plays a secondary role to diffusion weighted imaging and a peripheral zone lesion with an equivocal score of 3 on diffusion weighted imaging, a positive DCE-MRI upgrades overall lesion score from 3 to 4 (Fig. 4.8). However, it gains more importance in overall lesion scoring if image quality from diffusion weighted imaging is sub-optimal, and in detection of small cancers, and to aid in identifying benign causes of elevated PSA (Fig. 4.9).

Putting It Together: PI-RADS v2.1 Overall Assessment

PI-RADS v2.1 assessment uses a 5-point scale based on the probability that a combination of multiparametric MRI findings on T2 weighted, diffusion weighted imaging, and DCE correlates with the presence of a clinically significant cancer for each lesion in the prostate gland.

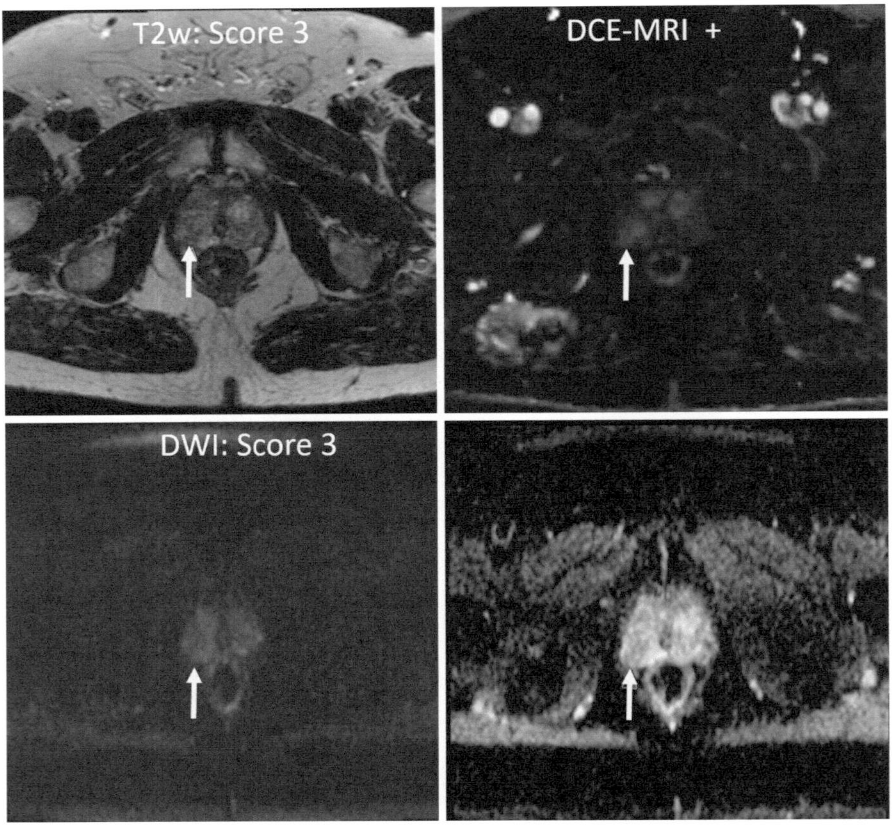

Fig. 4.8 Peripheral zone lesion upgrading with dynamic contrast enhanced (DCE)-MRI. Transverse T2 weighted image shows a focal dark lesion in left peripheral zone (arrow) which was scored 3 on diffusion weighted imaging (DWI). However, the lesion also shows early enhancement on subtracted DCE-MRI and thus overall lesion score was 4

Thus the overall PI-RADS v2.1 assessment categories are as follows:

- PI-RADS 1—Very low probability (clinically significant cancer is highly unlikely to be present)
- PI-RADS 2—Low probability (clinically significant cancer is unlikely to be present)
- PI-RADS 3—Intermediate probability (the presence of clinically significant cancer is equivocal) (Figs. 4.10 and 4.11)
- PI-RADS 4—High (clinically significant cancer is likely to be present) (Fig. 4.12)
- PI-RADS 5—Very high (clinically significant cancer is highly likely to be present) (Fig. 4.13)

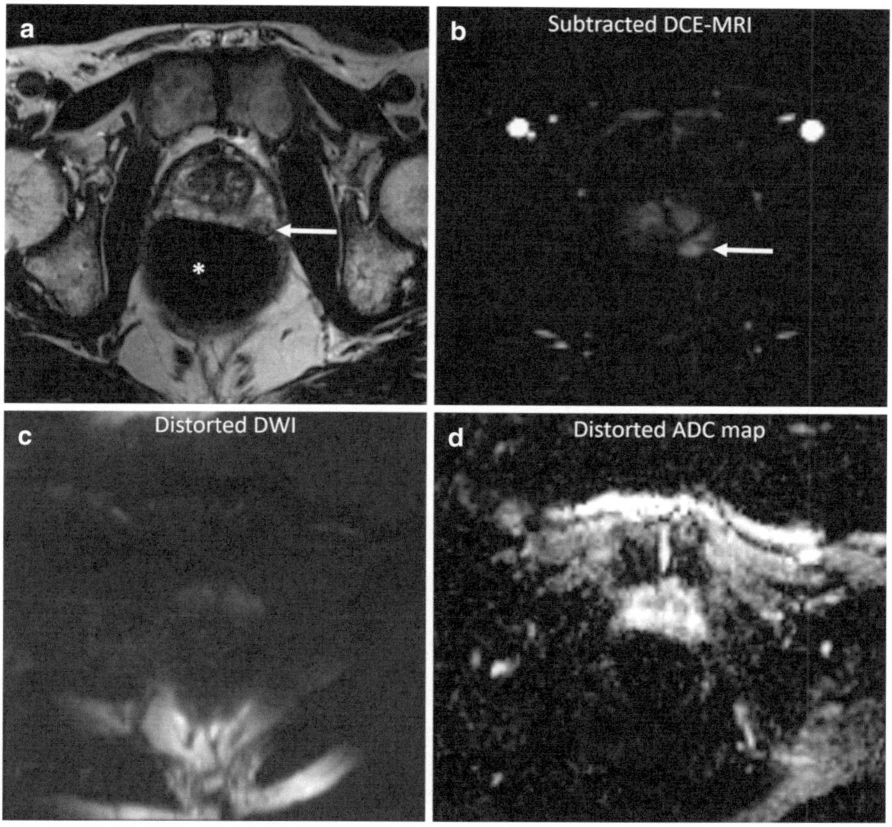

Fig. 4.9 Utility of dynamic contrast enhanced (DCE)-MRI in presence of distorted diffusion weighted imaging. Early enhancement (**b**) of a focal lesion seen on T2 weighted image (**a**) is suspicious for malignancy and upgrades overall lesion score from 3 to 4 while the diffusion weighted imaging (**c**) and the apparent diffusion coefficient map (**d**) are distorted

For peripheral zone, diffusion weighted imaging with apparent diffusion coefficient mapping is the primary/dominant sequence for scoring while DCE—MRI is the secondary/deciding sequence (Fig. 4.14). Thus a peripheral zone lesion with diffusion weighted imaging score of 3 is upgraded to 4 if DCE-MRI is positive (Fig. 4.8).

For transition zone, the T2 weighted sequence is the primary/dominant sequence for scoring while diffusion weighted imaging is the secondary/deciding sequence for both category 2 and 3 lesions on T2 weighted images (Fig. 4.15). Thus, if diffusion weighted imaging score is ≥ 4, a transition zone lesion with a T2 weighted score of 2 is upgraded to overall category 3. Similarly a lesion with T2 weighted score of 3 is upgraded to overall category 4 if diffusion weighted imaging score is 5 (Fig. 4.16) [9].

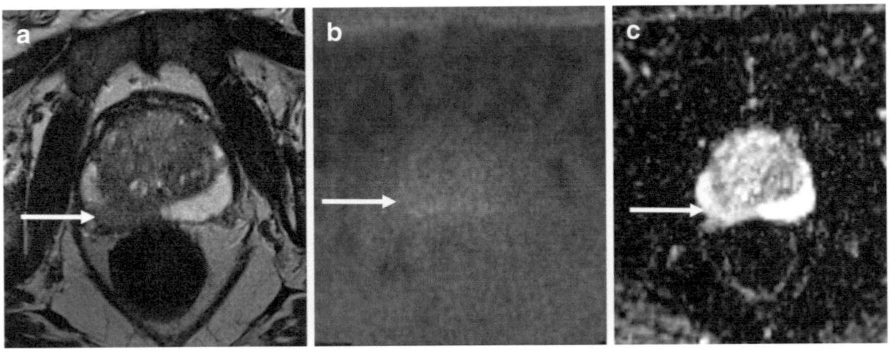

Fig. 4.10 PI-RADS 3 lesion in peripheral zone. T2 weighted image shows a lobar lesion with moderate low signal intensity (T2 weighted score 3). The lesion is isointense on diffusion weighted imaging (**b**) and shows mild decrease in signal on apparent diffusion coefficient (**c**) map (Diffusion weighted imaging score of 3). Hence overall PI-RADS score for the lesion is 3 and biopsy showed prostatitis

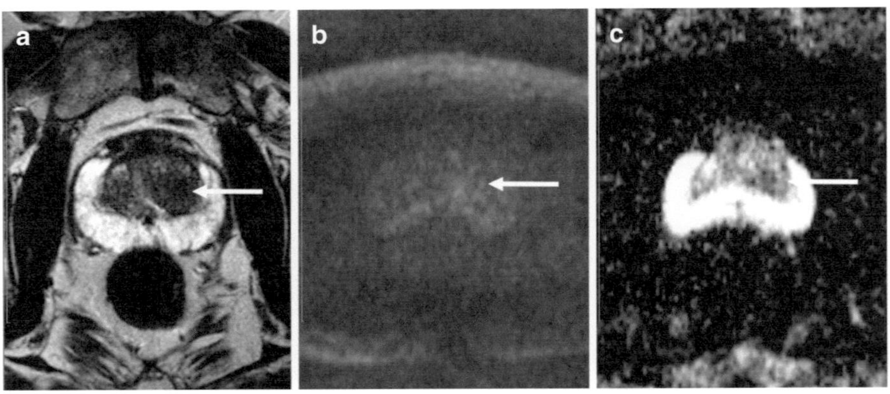

Fig. 4.11 PI-RADS 3 lesion in transition zone. T2 weighted image shows a lesion with obscured margins and low signal intensity in left posterior transition zone (T2 score 3). The lesion is isointense on diffusion weighted imaging (**b**) and shows a mild decrease in signal on apparent diffusion coefficient (**c**) map (Diffusion weighted imaging score of 3). Hence overall PI-RADS score for the lesion is 3

Overall PI-RADS v2 Assessment in Case of Inadequate Diffusion Weighted Imaging

As is evident from the scoring system, diffusion weighted imaging is the critical sequence for primary evaluation of peripheral zone lesions and for secondary evaluation of transition zone lesions with T2 weighted score of 2 and 3. Thus effort must be made to optimize the diffusion weighted imaging acquisition and get the best image quality, even if it requires repeating the sequence more than once during the scan. If after all attempts, diffusion weighted imaging yields inadequate image quality, this should be specifically mentioned in the report and scoring may be done on basis of T2 weighted images for both peripheral zone and transition zone lesions (Table 4.4) (Fig. 4.9).

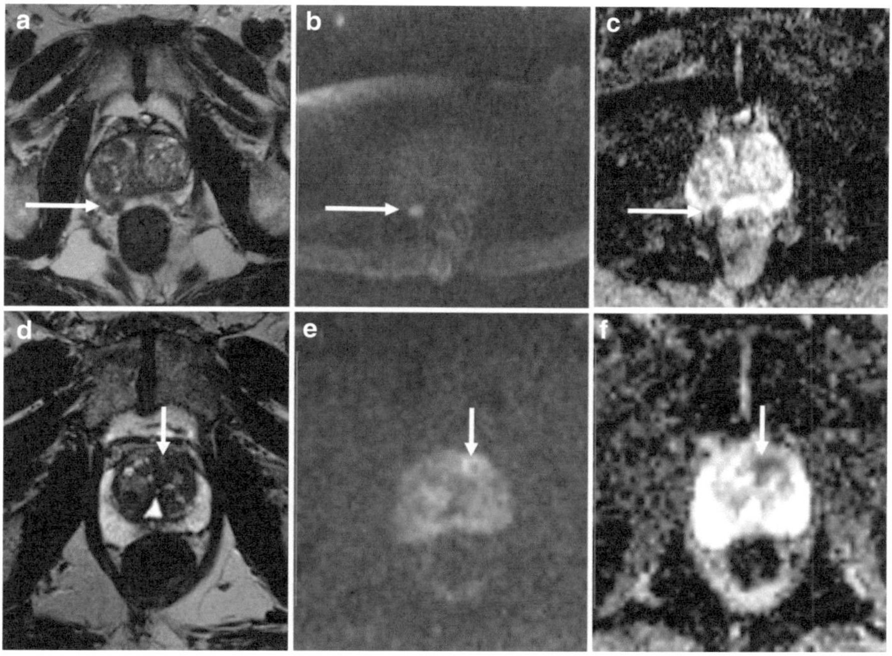

Fig. 4.12 PI-RADS 4 lesions in peripheral zone (**a–c**) and transition zone (**d–f**). PI-RADS 4 lesions are focal, markedly dark on T2 weighted images, show definite diffusion restriction and measure less than 1.5 cm in size

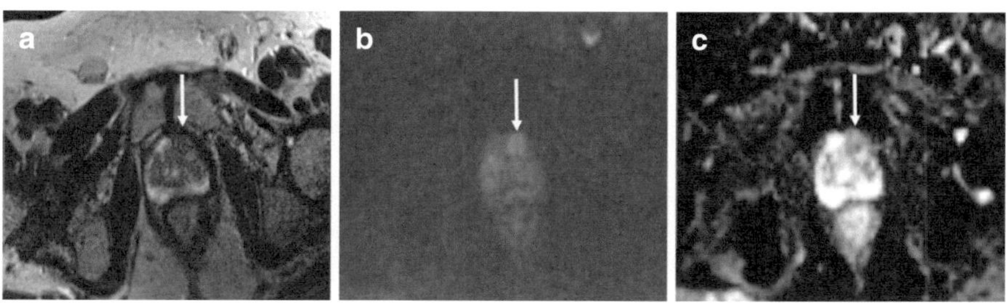

Fig. 4.13 PI-RADS 5 lesion in transition zone. Axial T2 weighted image shows a focal lesion with low signal intensity and diffusion restriction (**b**, **c**) and measuring more than 1.5 cm and thus overall scored as PI-RADS 5

Overall PI-RADS v2 Assessment for Peripheral Zone Lesions in Case of Non-contrast Biparametric MR Exam

Due to various reasons, it is possible that contrast is not administered during the MR exam and an entirely non-contrast MR exam may be performed. In case of such a biparametric exam, comprising of only T2 weighted and diffusion weighted imaging, the overall PI-RADS v2 category for peripheral zone lesions is entirely based

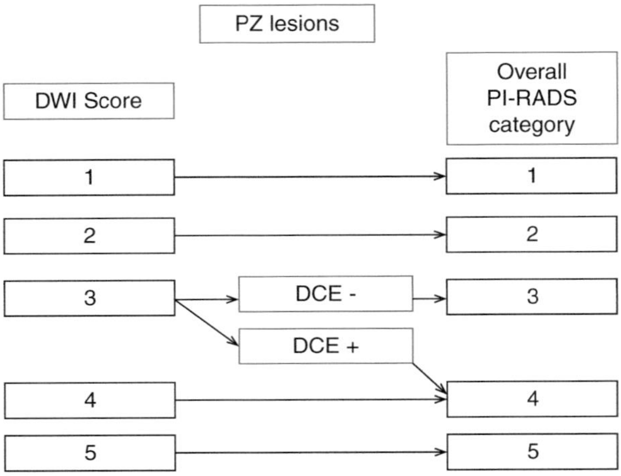

Fig. 4.14 Flowchart representing PI-RADS scoring system for peripheral zone lesions. *PZ* peripheral zone, *DWI* diffusion weighted imaging, *DCE* dynamic contrast enhanced

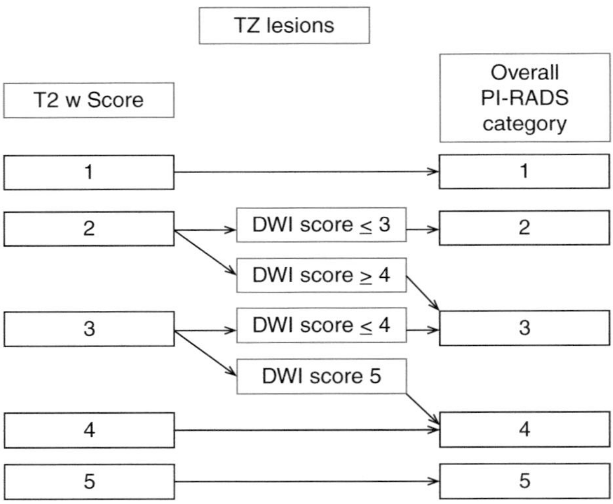

Fig. 4.15 Flowchart representing PI-RADS scoring system for transition zone lesions. *TZ* transition zone, *DWI* diffusion weighted imaging, *DCE* dynamic contrast enhanced

solely on the diffusion weighted imaging score. Thus a peripheral zone lesion with diffusion weighted imaging score of 3 is given an overall score of 3 in the absence of DCE-MRI for secondary decision-making.

For transition zone, since PI-RADS v2 evaluation is based only on T2 weighted and diffusion weighted imaging sequences, the lack of DCE-MRI does not alter the overall assessment.

Caveats in PI-RADS v2 Assessment and Updates in v2.1 Assessment

PI-RADS v2 acknowledged certain caveats when it comes to assessment of lesions and makes efforts to address them in the recent update. For example, some BPH nodules in the transition zone are not clearly encapsulated, and they may exhibit low

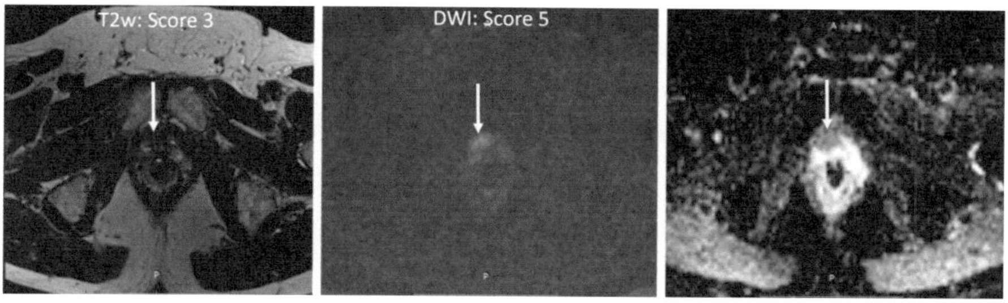

Fig. 4.16 Diffusion weighted imaging (DWI) upgrading a transition zone lesion. Axial T2 weighted image shows a lesion with moderately low signal intensity in anterior apical transition zone, measuring more than 1.5 cm. Based on T2 weighted image, the score for this lesion was 3. However, the lesion shows marked diffusion restriction (bright on high b-value DWI and very dark on corresponding apparent diffusion coefficient map) and scored 5 based on DWI. Thus overall score for the lesion is PI-RADS 5

Table 4.4 Overall PI-RADS v2 Assessment in case of inadequate diffusion weighted imaging

T2 weighted score	Diffusion weighted imaging	DCE-MRI	Overall PI-RADS v2 category
1	X	Any	1
2	X	Any	2
3	X	–	3
		+	4
4	X	Any	4
5	X	Any	5

signal intensity on apparent diffusion coefficient maps and increased signal intensity on high b-value diffusion weighted imaging. In the original v2 scoring system they would be considered overall Category 3 (T2 weighted score of 3, diffusion weighted score = 3), but now considered as overall Category 2 lesions (T2 weighted score = 2, diffusion weighted imaging score = 3).

Secondly, an encapsulated, circumscribed, round nodule with low signal intensity in the peripheral zone is likely a protruding BPH nodule, even if it is hypointense on apparent diffusion coefficient map and the PI-RADS Assessment Category for this finding should be 1 as per transition zone guidelines.

Third, since PI-RADS v2 assessment is individualized for peripheral zone and transition zone, it is important to correctly identify where the lesion is located. However, exact lesion localization may be confounded by distortion of normal anatomy due to BPH. Also, the central zone at the base of the prostate may be pushed or distorted by the enlarged transition zone and due to its low signal intensity on T2 weighted images, it might be mistaken for a transition zone cancer and subjected to unnecessary biopsy. Evaluation in all three planes and knowledge of normal anatomy at the base of prostate is helpful in avoiding mistaking a normal central zone for cancer. Similarly, the anterior fibromuscular stroma and anterior-apical regions of prostate represent potential areas where cancers may be hidden within the low signal intensity of normal anterior fibromuscular stroma. In such cases, diffusion weighted imaging is helpful and evidence of significant diffusion restriction can greatly help in overall scoring. These atypical locations are discussed in more detail in the Chap. 4.

MR Staging of Prostate Cancer

MRI is useful for local staging of prostate cancer, to differentiate between organ confined cancer ($\leq$ T2 disease) versus extraprostatic extension and/or seminal vesicle invasion ($\geq$ T3 disease). Anatomic T2 weighted images are the best sequence for local staging, complemented by T1 weighted imaging. diffusion weighted imaging and DCE-MRI are useful for assessment of seminal vescicle invasion, neurovascular bundle involvement and lymph node metastasis.

MR Criteria for Extra-Prostatic Extension [11, 12] (Figs. 4.17 **and** 4.18)

- Bulging prostatic contour
- Irregular/spiculated margin of prostate/capsular retraction
- Tumor-capsule interface >1 cm
- Encasement of neurovascular bundles by tumor/asymmetry in appearance of neurovascular bundle
- Obliteration of rectoprostatic angle/fat plane
- Direct invasion of tumor into bladder/rectum

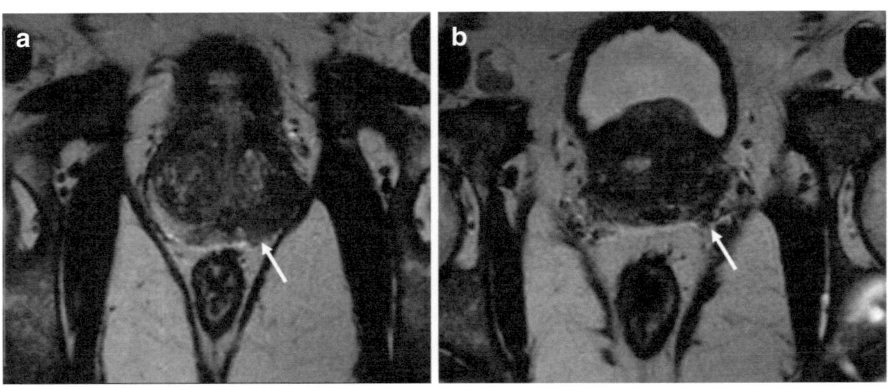

Fig. 4.17 Examples of extracapsular extension. (**a**) shows tumor with spiculated capsular margin, extension into periprostatic fat and tumor/capsule interface of more than 1.5 cm (**b**) shows asymmetrical appearance of neurovascular bundles with tumor abutting left neurovascular bundle (arrow)

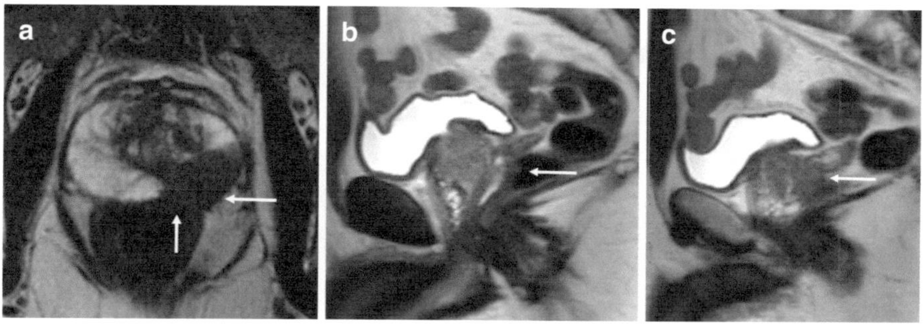

Fig. 4.18 Examples of extracapsular extension and potential rectal involvement. Along with tumor/capsular interface of more than 1.5 cm (**a**), there is also loss of fat plane with the rectum (**a**, **c**) suggestive of involvement of the rectum

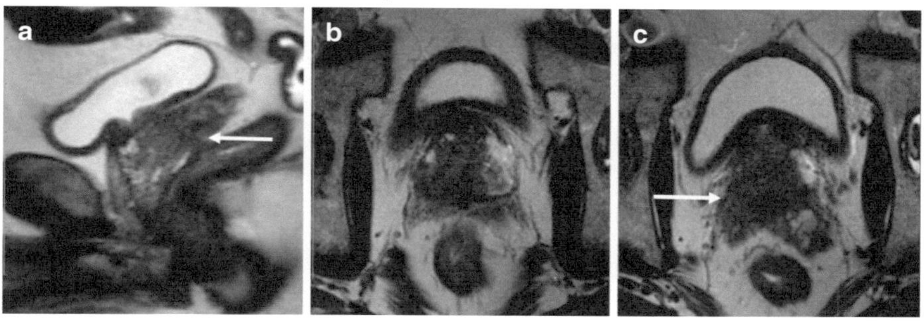

Fig. 4.19 Seminal vesicle invasion. Tumor at the base of prostate (**b**) shows direct extension into seminal vesicles (**c**) and loss of normal acute angle between seminal vesicle and prostate (arrow, **a**)

MR Criteria for Seminal Vesicle Invasion [11, 12] (Fig. 4.19)

- Low signal intensity of seminal vesicle with/without diffusion restriction/ abnormal enhancement along/within lumen of seminal vesicle
- Extension of tumor between prostate base and seminal vesicle with obliteration of normal angle between seminal vesicle and base of prostate (best seen on sagittal plane)
- Evidence of direct extension of tumor from base of prostate to seminal vesicle along ejaculatory duct
- Though less common, there can also be a metachronous tumor deposit within the seminal vesicle seen as a separate lesion on a T2 weighted image, distinct from another tumor focus within the prostate gland

The apical region of the prostate should be specifically evaluated for urethral involvement and for extraprostatic extension.

Lymph node assessment is mainly based on size criteria. Lymph nodes ≥8 mm in short axis diameter, with/without low single intensity or abnormal shapes are

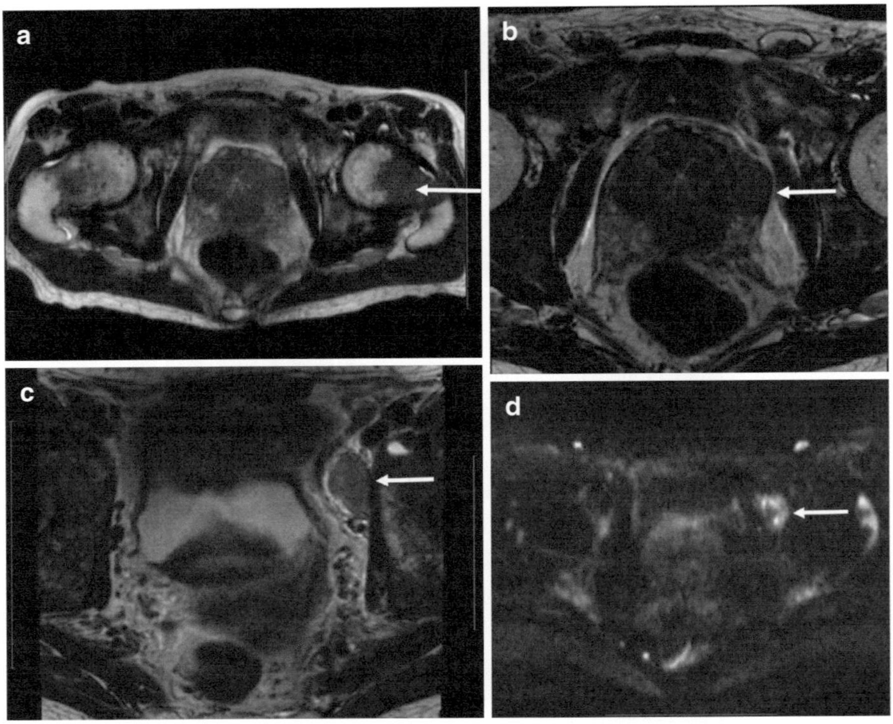

Fig. 4.20 Axial images of patient with metastatic Gleason 9 (5 + 4 = 9) show focal lesions in both femurs replacing normal bone marrow (arrow, **a**) and external iliac lymphadenopathy (arrow **c**). Malignant lymph nodes also show diffusion restriction, appearing bright on high b-value image (arrow, **d**)

suspicious for metastatic involvement. Abnormal contrast enhancement or marked diffusion restriction can be additionally helpful in detection (Fig. 4.20).

Nodal groups that should be evaluated include: common femoral, obturator, external iliac, internal iliac, common iliac, pararectal, presacral, paracaval, and para-aortic nodes to the level of the aortic bifurcation if included in large field of view images.

In addition, large field of view images should be assessed for presence of skeletal metastases and if present, should be mentioned in the report (Fig. 4.20).

Reporting Template and Mapping

To standardize reporting and facilitate easy communication between radiologist and urologists for further decision-making, PI-RADS v2 recommends using a reporting template and recommends visual mapping of the lesions. Examples of the template and the sector map from PI-RADS v2 are shown in Figs. 4.21 and 4.22.

Clinical Indication for MRI
Recent PSA level (ng/ml)

MRI Report

Prostate volume: Size must be measured as maximum transverse (T) x maximum anteroposterior (AP) x maximum longitudinal (L) diameter (cms)
Volume can be calculated as 0.52 x T x AP x L cm^3

Lesion reporting

Upto 4 lesions may be described, each assigned to a PIRADS category of 3, 4 or 5,
Index lesion must be identified. Index lesion refers to either lesion with highest overall category or with EPE

For every lesion:

- *Location* of lesion should be described with reference to sectors described in sector map and may also be visually mapped for easier understanding
- *Size* measured as largest diameter of the lesion in axial plane. If largest diamension of the lesion is seen on sagittal/coronal plane, then this diameter should be mentioned along with the plane. PZ lesions should be preferably measured on DWI while TZ lesions should be measured on T2w
- Signal characteristics on T2w/DWI with sequence scoring.
- EPE +/–, SVI +/–
- **Overall PI-RADS category**

Other findings (for staging): Suspicious lymph nodes, suspicious bone metastasis,

Other benign findings such as cysts may be reported to use as landmarks for targeted biopsies or to identify lesions on MR follow-up

Fig. 4.21 Recommended reporting template for reporting prostate MRI

Review and Limitations of PI-RADS v2

Since its release in 2015, various studies have assessed the diagnostic accuracy of PI-RADS v2 in detecting prostate cancer and a recent meta-analysis showed PI-RADS v2 to have a pooled sensitivity of 85% (78–91%) and pooled specificity of 71% (60–80%) for detection of all prostate cancer (Gleason grade 3+ 3 and above) [13]. In a head-to-head comparison between PI-RADS versions 1 and 2, v2 was shown to have a better diagnostic performance for transition zone lesions while v1 performed better in the peripheral zone [14]. In another study, PI-RADS v2 showed higher AUC (0.91) for detecting clinically significant cancers (Gleason 3+ 4 and above) and for experienced readers as compared to inexperienced readers [15]. The latest updates (v2.1) have been geared to further improve analysis of transition zone lesions. In the future, head to-head comparisons of PI-RADS v2 and v2.1 may better define the utility of MRI in detecting clinically significant cancers for both peripheral and transition zones using these revised guidelines.

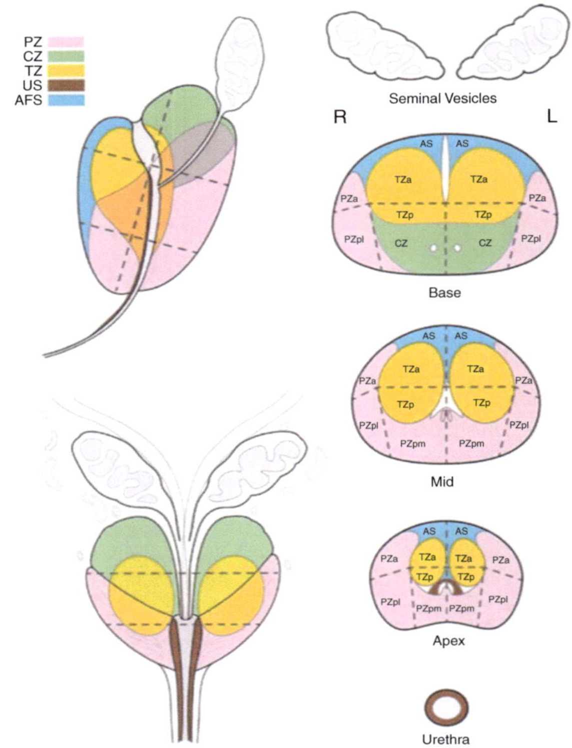

Total 39 sectors: 36 for Prostate, 2 for right and left seminal vesicles, 1 for external urethral sphincter

Right –Left division along line passing through urethra

Anterior-Posterior division along horizontal line through the middle of the gland.

Base. Mid-gland and apex is by rule of thirds in coronal/sagittal plane

Right and left perpheral zones (PZ) at prostate base, midgland, and apex are each subdivided into three sections: anterior (a), posterior mental (mp), and posterior lateral (pl)

Right and left transition zones (TZ) at prostate base, midgland, and apex are each subdivided into two sections: anterior (a), and posterior (p)

The central zone (CZ) is included in the prostate base around the ejaculatory ducts and is divided into right/left

The anterior fibromuscular stroma (AS) is divided into right/left at the prostate base, midgland, and apex

Fig. 4.22 Sector map for topographical location of lesions (PI-RADS v2 version). Using a sector map for reporting allows easier understanding between clinicians to understand location of lesion and plan intervention and therapy. *Note the PI-RADS v2.1 recognizes two additional sectors for the right and left posterior medial PZ at the base (PZpm), interposed between the central zone and the PZpl. Thus 41 sectors are now identified under PI-RADS v2.1compared to the 39 sectors under PI-RADS v2*

One of the current limitations of PI-RADS v2 is that inter-reader agreement is only moderate even for experienced readers [16–18] suggesting that further refinement in criteria is needed. While PI-RADS v2.1 makes descriptions more specific to decrease ambiguity, training of readers may be needed to ensure these updates can be reflected and implemented in clinical practice.

Another limitation is the lack of management recommendations, especially for PI-RADS category 3 lesions. Currently, PI-RADS category 3 lesions remain a gray-zone in terms of assessment and subsequent management. There is lack of sufficient inter-reader agreement on classifying a lesion as category 3. As shown by Purysko et al. [17], when a PI-RADSv2 assessment category ≥3 was considered positive, the agreement between readers was only fair to good, with lower agreement for transition zone lesions ($\kappa = 0.53$). On the other hand, when a PI-RADSv2 assessment category ≥4 was considered positive, the agreement was excellent overall and for both transition zone ($\kappa = 0.87$) and peripheral zone lesions ($\kappa = 0.91$). Secondly, Category 3 lesions have a very low yield for cancer (7–16%) [19, 20] when compared with MR-targeted biopsy results implying that most PI-RADS 3 lesions are being over-biopsied. Future refinements may include management guidelines for PI-RADS category 3 lesions to more accurately reflect current clinical practices [21].

Recent updates in PI-RADS v2.1 have re-evaluated the of role of DCE-MRI in evaluation prostate cancer and acknowledge the utility of a biparametric protocol for screening or risk-stratification of patients with elevated PSA as described in the next chapter [22, 23]. It is also hoped that the updates in PI-RADS v2.1 may decrease the number of unnecessary biopsies. Finally, current recommendations are entirely qualitative, with significant downplay of quantitative information that may be obtained from functional imaging sequences. However quantitative information from both relaxometry and apparent diffusion coefficient mapping may have significant added value [24]. While relaxometry is currently under research and reproducibility of apparent diffusion coefficient values remains an issue, future versions of PI-RADS may incorporate quantitative information in evaluation of prostate cancer. The last chapter discusses these potential future directions in greater detail.

References

1. Furlan A, Borhani AA, Westphalen AC. Multiparametric MR imaging of the prostate. Radiol Clin North Am. 2018;56:223. https://doi.org/10.1016/j.rcl.2017.10.005. [cited 2017 Dec 13].
2. Cruz M, Tsuda K, Narumi Y, Kuroiwa Y, Nose T, Kojima Y, et al. Characterization of low-intensity lesions in the peripheral zone of prostate on pre-biopsy endorectal coil MR imaging. Eur Radiol. 2002;12(2):357–65.
3. Mizuno R, Nakashima J, Mukai M, Ookita H, Nakagawa K, Oya M, et al. Maximum tumor diameter is a simple and valuable index associated with the local extent of disease in clinically localized prostate cancer. Int J Urol. 2006;13(7):951–5.
4. Tamada T, Sone T, Jo Y, Yamamoto A, Yamashita T, Egashira N, et al. Prostate cancer: relationships between postbiopsy hemorrhage and tumor detectability at MR diagnosis. Radiology. 2008;248(2):531–9.
5. Delongchamps NB, Rouanne M, Flam T, Beuvon F, Liberatore M, Zerbib M, et al. Multiparametric magnetic resonance imaging for the detection and localization of prostate

cancer: combination of T2-weighted, dynamic contrast-enhanced and diffusion-weighted imaging. BJU Int. 2011;107(9):1411–8.
6. Haider MA, van der Kwast TH, Tanguay J, Evans AJ, Hashmi A-T, Lockwood G, et al. Combined T2-weighted and diffusion-weighted MRI for localization of prostate cancer. Am J Roentgenol. 2007;189(2):323–8.
7. Hötker AM, Mazaheri Y, Aras Ö, Zheng J, Moskowitz CS, Gondo T, et al. Assessment of prostate cancer aggressiveness by use of the combination of quantitative DWI and dynamic contrast-enhanced MRI. AJR Am J Roentgenol. 2016;206(4):756–63.
8. Kitajima K, Kaji Y, Fukabori Y, Yoshida K, Suganuma N, Sugimura K. Prostate cancer detection with 3 T MRI: comparison of diffusion-weighted imaging and dynamic contrast-enhanced MRI in combination with T2-weighted imaging. J Magn Reson Imaging. 2010;31(3):625–31.
9. Turkbey B, Rosenkrantz AB, Haider MA, Padhani AR, Villeirs G, Macura KJ, et al. Prostate imaging reporting and data system version 2.1: 2019 update of prostate imaging reporting and data system version 2. Eur Urol. 2019 [cited 2019 Jun 27]. https://www.europeanurology.com/article/S0302-2838(19)30180-0/abstract.
10. Verma S, Turkbey B, Muradyan N, Rajesh A, Cornud F, Haider MA, et al. Overview of dynamic contrast-enhanced MRI in prostate cancer diagnosis and management. AJR Am J Roentgenol. 2012;198(6):1277–88.
11. Yu KK, Hricak H, Alagappan R, Chernoff DM, Bacchetti P, Zaloudek CJ. Detection of extracapsular extension of prostate carcinoma with endorectal and phased-array coil MR imaging: multivariate feature analysis. Radiology. 1997;202(3):697–702.
12. Hoeks CMA, Barentsz JO, Hambrock T, Yakar D, Somford DM, Heijmink SWTPJ, et al. Prostate cancer: multiparametric MR imaging for detection, localization, and staging. Radiology. 2011;261(1):46–66.
13. Zhang L, Tang M, Chen S, Lei X, Zhang X, Huan Y. A meta-analysis of use of Prostate Imaging Reporting and Data System Version 2 (PI-RADS V2) with multiparametric MR imaging for the detection of prostate cancer. Eur Radiol. 2017;27:5204.
14. Polanec S, Helbich TH, Bickel H, Pinker-Domenig K, Georg D, Shariat SF, et al. Head-to-head comparison of PI-RADS v2 and PI-RADS v1. Eur J Radiol. 2016;85(6):1125–31.
15. Kasel-Seibert M, Lehmann T, Aschenbach R, Guettler FV, Abubrig M, Grimm M-O, et al. Assessment of PI-RADS v2 for the detection of prostate cancer. Eur J Radiol. 2016;85(4):726–31.
16. Muller BG, Shih JH, Sankineni S, Marko J, Rais-Bahrami S, George AK, et al. Prostate cancer: interobserver agreement and accuracy with the revised prostate imaging reporting and data system at multiparametric MR imaging. Radiology. 2015;277(3):741–50.
17. Purysko AS, Bittencourt LK, Bullen JA, Mostardeiro TR, Herts BR, Klein EA. Accuracy and interobserver agreement for prostate imaging reporting and data system, version 2, for the characterization of lesions identified on multiparametric MRI of the prostate. AJR Am J Roentgenol. 2017;209(2):339–49.
18. Greer MD, Brown AM, Shih JH, Summers RM, Marko J, Law YM, et al. Accuracy and agreement of PI-RADSv2 for prostate cancer mpMRI: a multireader study. J Magn Reson Imaging. 2017;45(2):579–85.
19. Liddell H, Jyoti R, Haxhimolla HZ. mp-MRI prostate characterised PI-RADS 3 lesions are associated with a low risk of clinically significant prostate cancer - a retrospective review of 92 biopsied PI-RADS 3 lesions. Curr Urol. 2015;8(2):96–100.
20. Mertan FV, Greer MD, Shih JH, George AK, Kongnyuy M, Muthigi A, et al. Prospective evaluation of the prostate imaging reporting and data system version 2 for prostate cancer detection. J Urol. 2016;196(3):690–6.
21. Scialpi M, Martorana E, Aisa MC, Rondoni V, D'Andrea A, Bianchi G. Score 3 prostate lesions: a gray zone for PI-RADS v2. Turk J Urol. 2017 Sep;43(3):237–40.
22. Scialpi M, Martorana E, Aisa MC, Rondoni V, D'Andrea A, Brunese L. Abbreviated biparametric prostate MR Imaging: is it really an alternative to multiparametric MR imaging? Radiology. 2018;286(1):360–1.

23. Kuhl CK, Bruhn R, Krämer N, Nebelung S, Heidenreich A, Schrading S. Abbreviated biparametric prostate MR imaging in men with elevated prostate-specific antigen. Radiology. 2017;285(2):493–505.
24. Yu AC, Badve C, Ponsky LE, Pahwa S, Dastmalchian S, Rogers M, et al. Development of a combined MR fingerprinting and diffusion examination for prostate cancer. Radiology. 2017;283(3):729–38.

Biparametric MRI of Prostate: Can We Shorten the MR Imaging Protocol?

5

Verena Obmann, Ananya Panda, and Vikas Gulani

Introduction

According to the International Agency for Research on Cancer, annual incidence of cancer cases will be doubling by 2030 and prostate cancer is expected to be a major contributor [1]. As of 2018, prostate cancer accounts for 20% of all male cancer cases and 9% of cancer related deaths [2]. The ongoing challenges in the diagnosis and management of prostate cancer include identifying biologically significant disease at a stage while is still at a curative size and grade, while minimizing the detection of clinically insignificant cancers (Gleason score = 3 + 3 = 6) [3]. The widespread adoption of prostate specific antigen (PSA) as a screening tool led to a decrease in prostate cancer mortality [4]. However, there is concern that PSA screening has led to overdiagnosis and overtreatment of clinically insignificant prostate cancers. There is an ongoing need for improved prostate cancer screening tools to prevent both deaths related to aggressive prostate cancer and morbidity due to unnecessary treatment. Moreover, there has been rising concern over the morbidity and cost of over-diagnosis and overtreatment in men diagnosed with low risk, clinically non-significant disease (Gleason grade $\leq 3 + 4$) based on abnormal PSA level or abnormal DRE findings [5, 6]. Hence, a secondary screening diagnostic tool with a high negative predictive value for clinically significant cancer is desirable.

V. Obmann
Department of Diagnostic, Interventional and Pediatric Radiology (DIPR), Inselspital, Bern University Hospital, University of Bern, Bern, Switzerland
e-mail: verena.obmann@insel.ch

A. Panda
Department of Radiology, Mayo Clinic, Rochester, MN, USA
e-mail: panda.ananya@mayo.edu

V. Gulani (✉)
Fred Jenner Hodges Professor and Chair, Department of Radiology, University of Michigan, Ann Arbor, MI, USA
e-mail: vikasgulani@med.umich.edu

A. Panda et al. (eds.), *Reading MRI of the Prostate*,
https://doi.org/10.1007/978-3-319-99357-7_5

Multiparametric magnetic resonance imaging has emerged as an important tool in prostate cancer diagnosis and risk stratification with regard to the cancer aggressiveness [7, 8]. Depending on patient selection, it has a negative predictive value (NPV) of 63–98% [9] and it has been demonstrated that multiparametric MRI could reduce more than a quarter (27%) of unnecessary biopsies [8]. Thus, there is an increasing number of voices supporting consideration of pre-biopsy MRI in all men undergoing prostate biopsy [10]. Unfortunately, multiparametric MRI as a screening tool for prostate cancer is often seen as cost- and time-prohibitive due to the long scan times, patient discomfort associated with long MRI scans and the added cost of intravenous contrast.

Rationale for a Shortened Biparametric Protocol

As described in prior chapters, multiparametric MRI combines T2 weighted (T2w), diffusion weighted imaging (DWI) with apparent diffusion coefficient mapping and dynamic contrast enhanced (DCE) imaging. Evaluation and reporting is based on the standards of the Prostate Imaging Reporting and Data System (PI-RADS) version 2.1 [11]. In PI-RADS version 2.1, T2 weighted- and diffusion weighted imaging sequences are key in determining the appropriate PI-RADS score while dynamic contrast enhanced imaging only serves as a modifier to upgrade peripheral zone lesions from PI-RADS Category 3 to Category 4 in the presence of early preferential enhancement. Following the PI-RADS guidelines there is no role for dynamic contrast enhanced imaging in the transition zone. Especially in settings where a Category 3 lesion would also be biopsied, it is thus logical that a biparametric MR imaging protocol consisting of T2 weighted imaging and diffusion weighted imaging may be sufficient for detecting clinical significant prostate cancer and risk stratification in patients while saving costs and time, and multiple groups have proposed and explored this route (Fig. 5.1).

Representative MRI Protocols: Biparametric vs. Multiparametric

Representative protocols for biparametric-MRI and multiparametric MRI are shown in Fig. 5.1. Biparametric-MRI generally consists of single shot (SS) T2 weighted images in different planes, an axial high resolution T2 weighted turbo spin echo (TSE) acquisition and diffusion weighted imaging with apparent diffusion coefficient mapping. It thus omits the injection of intravenous gadolinium but also reduces the number and extent of further characterizing T2 weighted and T1 weighted images (Fig. 5.2).

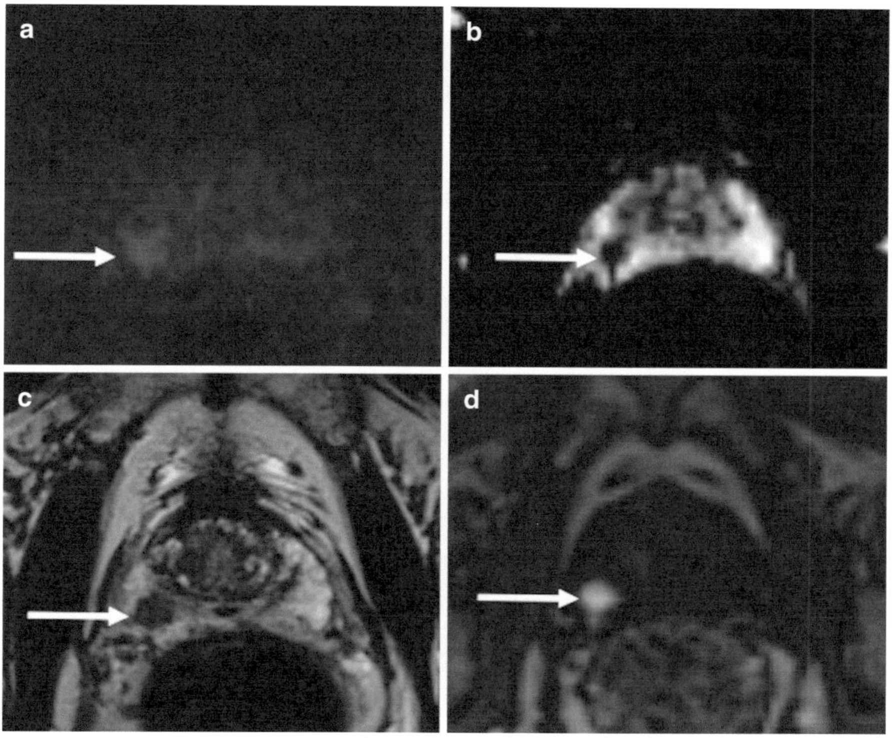

Fig. 5.1 Patient example demonstrating sequence overview differentiating biparametric from multiparametric MRI protocols. Diffusion weighted image (**a**) and apparent diffusion coefficient map (**b**) show focal diffusion restriction in the right peripheral zone at the base (arrow) with decreased apparent diffusion coefficient value (0.77×10^{-3} mm/s^2). Corresponding T2 weighted sequence (**c**) shows a 10 mm hypointense focal lesion. Based on biparametric image evaluation, the lesion is PI-RADS category 4. Although there is preferential early enhancement of the lesion (**d**), the dynamic contrast enhanced image is of no additional diagnostic value in this PI-RADS Category 4 lesion. Biopsy of the lesion revealed prostate cancer with a Gleason Score of 4 + 3 = 7

Advantages Using a Biparametric Protocol

Time Savings Using a Biparametric Protocol

The time slot for traditional multiparametric prostate MRI exam is typically approximately 45 min while the biparametric protocol achieves diagnostic accuracy in approximately a third of the table time without the use of a contrast agent. Using more recent imaging techniques such as simultaneous multislice imaging for diffusion imaging (DW-EPISMS) imaging time for a biparametric protocol can be shortened to as low as 5 min [12].

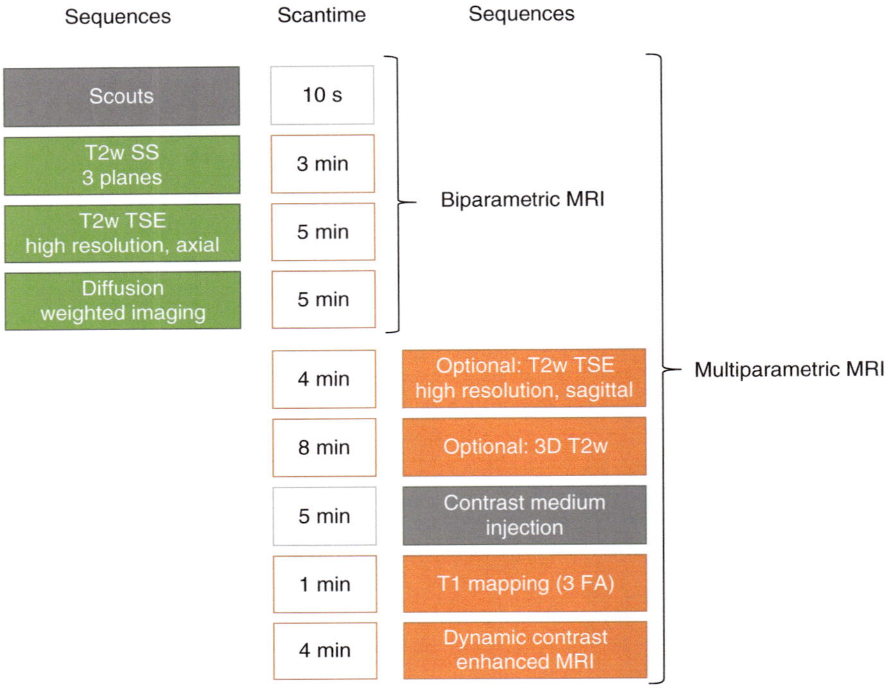

Fig. 5.2 Sequence overview differentiating biparametric from multiparametric MRI protocols. Biparametric-MRI typically consists of three sequences as shown in the green boxes: T2 weighted single shot acquisition for anatomical orientation (number of planes varies between institutions), a high resolution axial turbo spin echo sequence for lesion detection and characterization, as well as axial diffusion weighted imaging with apparent diffusion coefficient mapping. For the single shot T2 weighted sequences, the authors recommend all three planes (axial, coronal, sagittal) because the time expenditure is minimal and can help orient the urologist or provide information about extension of tumor. Multiparametric-MRI contains additional dynamic contrast enhanced imaging including T1 mapping which is needed for the quantification of perfusion parameters. Further high resolution or 3D T2 weighted sequences are part of the full multiparametric protocol, especially in the setting of staging and treatment planning. *T2w* T2 weighted, *SS* single shot, *TSE* turbo spin echo, *IV* intravenous, *MRI* magnetic resonance imaging, *FA* flip angle, *DCE* dynamic contrast enhanced

No Need for Intravenous Contrast Agents

Many men may have repeated (prostate and other) MRIs over their lifetimes. Given concerns about gadolinium deposition, current recommendations suggest that gadolinium use should be limited to settings where it is necessary for diagnosis, and this consideration may also factor into the use of this non-contrast protocol [13]. In 2017 the Food and Drug Administration (FDA) issued a new class warning and now mandates that patients receive proper counseling on this matter before receiving a gadolinium contrast agent [14]. A biparametric prostate MRI protocol without the need of intravenous gadolinium contrast agent injection is thus potentially useful in this screening setting, where patients may receive multiple exams over their lifetimes, and the benefit in image interpretation is minimal, at least according to current, PI-RADS V2.1 criteria. The downsides of a complete exam include the need for the IV gadolinium injection, expended time (needle placement, interruption of the exam to hook up the line and inject), and cost (about $100 material costs per scan).

Cost Savings Using a Biparametric Protocol

It further has also been shown through decision analysis models that such a biparametric protocol can be cost effective in clinical practice in a variety of settings [15–17]. As MRI finds more wide-spread adoption and implementation in the workflow of prostate cancer detection, even prior to first biopsy, it is imperative to be cost-conscious to allow for wider public health reach of benefit. As such, the use of biparametric protocol could significantly improve patient access while limiting many of the financial and time constraints institutions face with traditional multiparametric-MRI [18].

Diagnostic Accuracy Using a Biparametric Protocol

Diagnostic Accuracy Compared to mp-MRI

Several studies have compared a "biparametric reading session" out of a full multiparametric MRI protocol with the results of the latter in biopsy-naïve men [12, 19, 20] as well as in the setting of tumor recurrence assessment after therapy [21]. All showed that biparametric-MRI and multiparametric-MRI had similar or even higher [22] diagnostic accuracy as the full exam, but that biparametric-MRI has the advantage of being shorter and cheaper. In a meta-analysis by Woo et al. that included 20 studies with a head to head comparison of biparametric-MRI and multiparametric-MRI, both biparametric MRI and multiparametric-MRI had similar sensitivities of 74% and 76% and specificities of 90% and 89% respectively [23]. By including further articles (total of 33 studies), Niu et al. found a slightly higher sensitivity for multiparametric-MRI (85% [95% CI: 0.78–0.83]) compared to biparametric-MRI (80% [95% CI: 0.71–0.9]) [24]. However, if examining only the diagnostic accuracy for clinically significant cancer, both protocols perform similarly, with an incremental value for diagnostic accuracy of up to 3% in peripheral zone and no additional value in the detection of clinically significant transition zone cancer [25, 26].

Diagnostic Accuracy for Clinical Significant Cancer

Using a biparametric approach and thus omitting dynamic contrast enhanced imaging means potentially less information. It thus is important that if a MRI study is negative that there are as few as possible patients with cancer (false negative) or in other words, a high negative predictive value is desirable to prevent undertreatment. Obmann et al. [27] demonstrated a negative predictive value of the biparametric-MRI protocol of 96% for a modified PI-RADS score of ≥3 for clinically significant prostate cancer in a prospective study design. Here a modified PI-RADS score represents a score calculated similarly to the PI-RADS V2 guidelines, but omitting the dynamic contrast enhanced imaging component of the score. Similar results were shown by Boesen et al. (negative predictive value 97%) [28]. A low false positive rate is desirable to avoid unnecessary biopsies, increased costs, patient anxiety, over treatment in case of insignificant cancer.

Potential Drawbacks/Challenges of Biparametric-MRI

Loss of Potential Upgrade from PI-RADS Category 3 to 4 in the Peripheral Zone

An implicit trade-off in the biparametric approach is the loss of ability to potentially upgrade a Category 3 lesion to a Category 4 in the peripheral zone and thus a higher number of PI-RADS 3 lesions [29]. The importance of this tradeoff depends greatly on how the management of these lesions is approached at an institution. If the adopted approach is that all Category 3 or higher lesions are to be biopsied (the approach at our Institution), then there is no clinical consequence to a biparametric approach, as Category 3 and Category 4 lesions are both considered "biopsy" lesions. However, if the adopted approach involves not biopsying some or all of Category 3 lesions based on risk stratification, then the distinction between Category 3 and 4 has the potential to be clinically significant. Transition zone lesions would still not be affected by this biparametric approach, as dynamic contrast enhanced imaging plays no role in present PI-RADS guidelines, for categorizing these lesions. Similarly, patients with a higher suspicion of synchronous lesion would also still go to biopsy. If a decision is made to call back patients needing a dynamic contrast enhanced imaging stratification to make a biopsy decision, 20% of patients examined with a biparametric protocol could require additional dynamic contrast enhanced evaluation if an institution chooses to not biopsy Category 3 lesions as shown by Obmann et al. [27]. Of course, if the pretest suspicion of cancer is high in a subset of this group and thus a biopsy would be indicated regardless of dynamic contrast enhanced imaging score, then the fraction needing to be recalled would be lower.

Influence on Inter-Reader Agreement

Another potential drawback is the influence of biparamteric protocols on inter-reader agreement. It is known that the inter-reader agreement of multiparametric-MRI studies using PI-RADS v2 is only moderate to good, as shown in several studies (Muller et al. [30], $k = 0.37–0.45$, Rosenkrantz et al. [31], $k = 0.51–0.59$, or Greer et al. [32], index of specific agreement (ISA) 59% and 85%). A more recent study even demonstrated only low to moderate overall inter-reader agreement with lower agreement rates for T2 weighted and diffusion weighted imaging compared to the image evaluation of a full multiparametric-MRI protocol [33]. Thus the choice of reader could influence the results of a biparametric-MRI exam, though this is a drawback shared with the multiparametric-MRI as well.

Heterogeneity in Image Acquisition and Image Quality

Further, there is a lack of standardization and impacted image quality of diffusion weighted imaging. This leads to frequent artefacts and image distortion, especially in the presence of rectal gas or hip implants. The lack of standardization manifests in various protocols with different b-values used. There is a lot of variation in the number of b values as well as the highest b-value used among different institutions. Guidelines recommend a highest b-value of at least 1400 s/mm^2, or up to 2000 s/mm^2 if the signal-to-noise ratio remains adequate or alternatively by utilizing calculated high b-value images. On images with a high b-value ($\geq$1400 s/mm^2), the signal intensity of the normal prostate tissue is low, whereas the signal intensity of prostate cancer is high, representing restricted diffusion. However, as the b-value increases, the signal-to-noise ratio decreases, so that selection of the optimum high b-value may depend on magnetic field strength, software, and manufacturer [24]. Further, if the diffusion weighted imaging exam is corrupted by artifact, the reader may be left to utilize only T2 weighted images, which is a limitation of the biparametric-MRI examination not faced in an multiparametric-MRI setting where dynamic contrast enhanced imaging can serve as a backup sequence at least for peripheral zone lesions.

Potential Recall Exams in Certain Patients

Biparametric-MRI protocols are designed for a fast exam to triage between patients without and with clinical significant prostate cancer. As explained beforehand, this can save tremendous amount of time and healthcare costs and increase availability of prostate MRI for more men. However, since biparametric-MRI protocols are optimized for the detection of prostate cancer but not tested yet for staging, treatment planning or monitoring, there is a potential risk of a need for repeat exams with biparametric-MRI in those patients if more precise information is requested for patient treatment. For those patients pathways should be developed, i.e. using multiparametric-MRI in dedicated treatment planning studies, active surveillance or in very high risk patients with significantly high PSA >20 ng/mL, symptoms suggesting prostate cancer or a clinical T3/T4 stage [34]. Similarly, the risk of clinically significant cancer might be better estimated by using the risk calculator by the Prostate Cancer Research Foundation ("Stichting Wetenschappelijk Onderzoek Prostaatkanker", SWOP) instead of PSA or based on several epidemiological factors such as age, family history, genetic predisposition, race black and obesity [35]. This may allow better triage into the biparametric-MRI and multiparametric-MRI diagnostic pathways.

Summary/Conclusion

Biparametric-MRI can detect and localize prostate cancer. It may be argued that both PI-RADS 3 and 4 lesions require further attention regardless, and many urologists prefer to biopsy all lesions with PI-RADS ≥3. Hence, the effect of dynamic contrast enhanced imaging may not be critical and thus a biparametric-MRI pathway may be ideal in many settings for the right patients. Biparametric-MRI protocols can be implemented in clinical practice and utilized as a quick noninvasive test for triaging the multitude of men that need further workup based on a modified PI-RADS scoring system, from those with a very low probability of clinically significant cancer.

References

1. Bray F, Jemal A, Grey N, Ferlay J, Forman D. Global cancer transitions according to the Human Development Index (2008-2030): a population-based study. Lancet Oncol. 2012;13(8):790–801.
2. Siegel RL, Miller KD, Jemal A. Cancer statistics, 2018. CA Cancer J Clin. 2018;68(1):7–30.
3. Kozlowski P, Chang SD, Jones EC, Goldenberg SL. Assessment of the need for DCE MRI in the detection of dominant lesions in the whole gland: correlation between histology and MRI of prostate cancer. NMR Biomed. 2018;31(3):e3882.
4. Merrill RM, Stephenson RA. Trends in mortality rates in patients with prostate cancer during the era of prostate specific antigen screening. J Urol. 2000;163(2):503–10.
5. Loeb S, Bjurlin MA, Nicholson J, Tammela TL, Penson DF, Carter HB, et al. Overdiagnosis and overtreatment of prostate cancer. Eur Urol. 2014;65(6):1046–55.
6. Mariotto AB, Robin Yabroff K, Shao Y, Feuer EJ, Brown ML. Projections of the cost of cancer care in the United States: 2010–2020. J Natl Cancer Inst. 2011;103(2):117–28.
7. Abd-Alazeez M, Ahmed HU, Arya M, Charman SC, Anastasiadis E, Freeman A, et al. The accuracy of multiparametric MRI in men with negative biopsy and elevated PSA level—can it rule out clinically significant prostate cancer? Urol Oncol. 2014;32(1):45.e17–22.
8. Ahmed HU, El-Shater Bosaily A, Brown LC, Gabe R, Kaplan R, Parmar MK, et al. Diagnostic accuracy of multi-parametric MRI and TRUS biopsy in prostate cancer (PROMIS): a paired validating confirmatory study. Lancet. 2017;389(10071):815–22.
9. Futterer JJ, Briganti A, De Visschere P, Emberton M, Giannarini G, Kirkham A, et al. Can clinically significant prostate cancer be detected with multiparametric magnetic resonance imaging? A systematic review of the literature. Eur Urol. 2015;68(6):1045–53.
10. Meng X, Rosenkrantz AB, Mendhiratta N, Fenstermaker M, Huang R, Wysock JS, et al. Relationship between prebiopsy multiparametric magnetic resonance imaging (MRI), biopsy indication, and MRI-ultrasound fusion-targeted prostate biopsy outcomes. Eur Urol. 2016;69(3):512–7.
11. Weinreb JC, Barentsz JO, Choyke PL, Cornud F, Haider MA, Macura KJ, et al. PI-RADS prostate imaging - reporting and data system: 2015, version 2. Eur Urol. 2016;69(1):16–40.
12. Weiss J, Martirosian P, Notohamiprodjo M, Kaufmann S, Othman AE, Grosse U, et al. Implementation of a 5-minute magnetic resonance imaging screening protocol for prostate cancer in men with elevated prostate-specific antigen before biopsy. Investig Radiol. 2018;53(3):186–90.
13. Gulani V, Calamante F, Shellock FG, Kanal E, Reeder SB. Gadolinium deposition in the brain: summary of evidence and recommendations. Lancet Neurol. 2017;16(7):564–70.
14. Brief Fi. FDA requires new class warning and additional research on retention in the body of gadolinium from gadolinium-based contrast agents used in magnetic resonance imaging; 2017.

15. Cerantola Y, Dragomir A, Tanguay S, Bladou F, Aprikian A, Kassouf W. Cost-effectiveness of multiparametric magnetic resonance imaging and targeted biopsy in diagnosing prostate cancer. Urol Oncol. 2016;34(3):119.e1–9.
16. Pahwa S, Schiltz NK, Ponsky LE, Lu Z, Griswold MA, Gulani V. Cost-effectiveness of MR Imaging-guided strategies for detection of prostate cancer in biopsy-naive men. Radiology. 2017;285(1):157–66.
17. Faria R, Soares MO, Spackman E, Ahmed HU, Brown LC, Kaplan R, et al. Optimising the diagnosis of prostate cancer in the era of multiparametric magnetic resonance imaging: a cost-effectiveness analysis based on the Prostate MR Imaging Study (PROMIS). Eur Urol. 2017;73:23.
18. Sherrer RL, Glaser ZA, Gordetsky JB, Nix JW, Porter KK, Rais-Bahrami S. Comparison of biparametric MRI to full multiparametric MRI for detection of clinically significant prostate cancer. Prostate Cancer Prostatic Dis. 2019;22:331.
19. Di Campli E, Delli Pizzi A, Seccia B, Cianci R, d'Annibale M, Colasante A, et al. Diagnostic accuracy of biparametric vs multiparametric MRI in clinically significant prostate cancer: comparison between readers with different experience. Eur J Radiol. 2018;101:17–23.
20. Kuhl CK, Bruhn R, Kramer N, Nebelung S, Heidenreich A, Schrading S. Abbreviated biparametric prostate MR imaging in men with elevated prostate-specific antigen. Radiology. 2017;285(2):493–505.
21. Lotte R, Lafourcade A, Mozer P, Conort P, Barret E, Comperat E, et al. Multiparametric MRI for suspected recurrent prostate cancer after HIFU: is DCE still needed? Eur Radiol. 2018;28:3760.
22. De Visschere P, Lumen N, Ost P, Decaestecker K, Pattyn E, Villeirs G. Dynamic contrast-enhanced imaging has limited added value over T2-weighted imaging and diffusion-weighted imaging when using PI-RADSv2 for diagnosis of clinically significant prostate cancer in patients with elevated PSA. Clin Radiol. 2017;72(1):23–32.
23. Woo S, Suh CH, Kim SY, Cho JY, Kim SH, Moon MH. Head-to-head comparison between biparametric and multiparametric MRI for the diagnosis of prostate cancer: a systematic review and meta-analysis. AJR Am J Roentgenol. 2018;211(5):W226–w41.
24. Niu XK, Chen XH, Chen ZF, Chen L, Li J, Peng T. Diagnostic performance of biparametric MRI for detection of prostate cancer: a systematic review and meta-analysis. AJR Am J Roentgenol. 2018;211(2):369–78.
25. Vargas HA, Hotker AM, Goldman DA, Moskowitz CS, Gondo T, Matsumoto K, et al. Updated prostate imaging reporting and data system (PIRADS v2) recommendations for the detection of clinically significant prostate cancer using multiparametric MRI: critical evaluation using whole-mount pathology as standard of reference. Eur Radiol. 2016;26(6):1606–12.
26. Barth BK, Visschere PJLD, Cornelius A, Nicolau C, Vargas HA, Eberli D, et al. Detection of clinically significant prostate cancer: short dual–pulse sequence versus standard multiparametric MR imaging—a multireader study. Radiology. 2017;284(3):725–36.
27. Obmann VC, Pahwa S, Tabayayong W, Jiang Y, O'Connor G, Dastmalchian S, et al. Diagnostic accuracy of a rapid biparametric MRI protocol for detection of histologically proven prostate cancer. Urology. 2018;122:133–8.
28. Boesen L, Nørgaard N, Løgager V, et al. Assessment of the diagnostic accuracy of biparametric magnetic resonance imaging for prostate cancer in biopsy-naive men: the biparametric mri for detection of prostate cancer (bidoc) study. JAMA Netw Open. 2018;1(2):e180219.
29. Junker D, Steinkohl F, Fritz V, Bektic J, Tokas T, Aigner F, et al. Comparison of multiparametric and biparametric MRI of the prostate: are gadolinium-based contrast agents needed for routine examinations? World J Urol. 2019;37:691.
30. Muller BG, Shih JH, Sankineni S, Marko J, Rais-Bahrami S, George AK, et al. Prostate cancer: interobserver agreement and accuracy with the revised prostate imaging reporting and data system at multiparametric MR imaging. Radiology. 2015;277(3):741–50.
31. Rosenkrantz AB, Ginocchio LA, Cornfeld D, Froemming AT, Gupta RT, Turkbey B, et al. Interobserver reproducibility of the PI-RADS version 2 lexicon: a multicenter study of six experienced prostate radiologists. Radiology. 2016;280(3):793–804.

32. Greer MD, Brown AM, Shih JH, Summers RM, Marko J, Law YM, et al. Accuracy and agreement of PIRADSv2 for prostate cancer mpMRI: a multireader study. J Magn Reson Imaging. 2017;45(2):579–85.
33. Smith CP, Harmon SA, Barrett T, Bittencourt LK, Law YM, Shebel H, et al. Intra- and interreader reproducibility of PI-RADSv2: a multireader study. J Magn Reson Imaging. 2019;49:1694.
34. Van Nieuwenhove S, Saussez TP, Thiry S, Trefois P, Annet L, Michoux N, et al. Prospective comparison of a fast 1.5-T biparametric with the 3.0-T multiparametric ESUR magnetic resonance imaging protocol as a triage test for men at risk of prostate cancer. BJU Int. 2019;123:411.
35. Pernar CH, Ebot EM, Wilson KM, Mucci LA. The epidemiology of prostate cancer. Cold Spring Harb Perspect Med. 2018;8(12):a030361.

MRI Appearance of Prostate Cancers in Locations Posing Diagnostic or Biopsy Challenges

6

Ananya Panda and Vikas Gulani

Prostate cancer affects the peripheral zone more commonly than the transition zone, with 70% of prostate cancer arising from the peripheral zone, 25% of cancers in the transition zone and 5% in the central zone. Cancers outside the peripheral zone can often be missed due to their lower incidence, and relative lack of familiarity with the appearances of these non-peripheral zone cancers. In addition, since both central zone and anterior fibromuscular stroma are dark on T2 weighted images and anatomy is often distorted by an enlarged transition zone, it is harder to detect cancers in these locations. This chapter serves as a guide for evaluation of prostate cancers in diagnostically challenging locations atypical.

Peripheral Zone

Distal Apical Tumor The distal apical region refers to the distal 6 mm of the prostate (near the inferior tip). While the peripheral zone comprises a large portion of the distal apex and distal apical tumors have the same signal characteristics as rest of peripheral zone tumors, these can often be missed unless specifically searched for, on MRI [1]. In addition, these tumors can be missed on standard transrectal ultrasound (TRUS) guided biopsy as the sampling may miss the apex [2, 3], and thus a transperineal or image-guided/targeted biopsy is sometimes helpful [4] (Figs. 6.1 and 6.2).

A. Panda
Department of Radiology, Mayo Clinic, Rochester, MN, USA
e-mail: panda.ananya@mayo.edu

V. Gulani (✉)
Fred Jenner Hodges Professor and Chair, Department of Radiology, University of Michigan, Ann Arbor, MI, USA
e-mail: vikasgulani@med.umich.edu

A. Panda et al. (eds.), *Reading MRI of the Prostate*,
https://doi.org/10.1007/978-3-319-99357-7_6

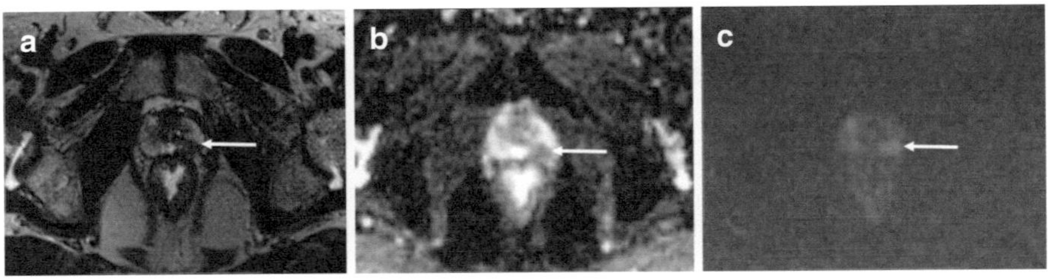

Fig. 6.1 Tumor in periapical peripheral zone. Axial T2 weighted image shows a focal lesion in left peripheral zone at the apex (**a**) with diffusion restriction (**b**, **c**). Although the appearance of tumor is typical, the distal location can cause it to be overlooked

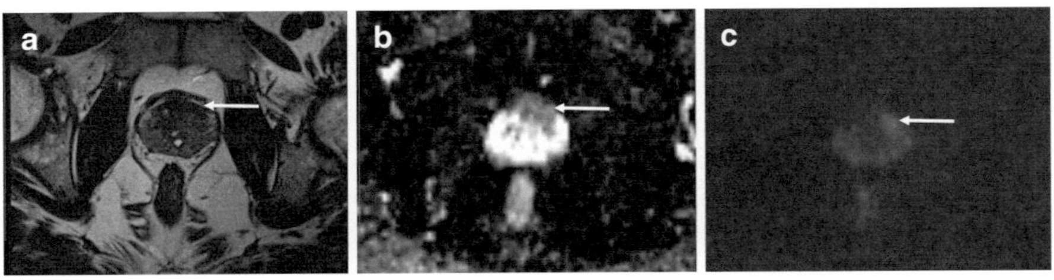

Fig. 6.2 Tumor in periapical transition zone. Axial T2 weighted image shows a large focal lesion in anterior apical transition (**a**) with diffusion restriction (**b**, **c**). The distal location and the dark signal of the background transition zone can cause the tumor to be missed on T2 weighted image. In such cases, diffusion restriction is helpful in detection

Subcapsular Crescentic Tumor A small crescentic tumor abutting the outer capsule has a high probability of extraprostatic extension, despite its small size. However, this can often be mistaken for thickening of the outer capsule. Diffusion weighted imaging with apparent diffusion coefficient mapping and dynamic contrast enhanced-MRI can help in detection of tumor in this location either due to presence of diffusion restriction with reduced apparent diffusion coefficient or focal early enhancement [5] (Fig. 6.3).

Diffuse Infiltrative Tumors While a typical peripheral zone tumor is a focus or a mass, at times tumors can be diffusely infiltrative without forming a distinct mass. These tumors are often low-grade (Gleason grade 3 + 3) tumors and have sparse cellularity admixed with normal prostate tissue [6]. Due to their relatively lower cellularity, they can be difficult to identify or invisible on mpMRI despite using high-resolution T2 weighted and diffusion weighted imaging [5] (Fig. 6.4).

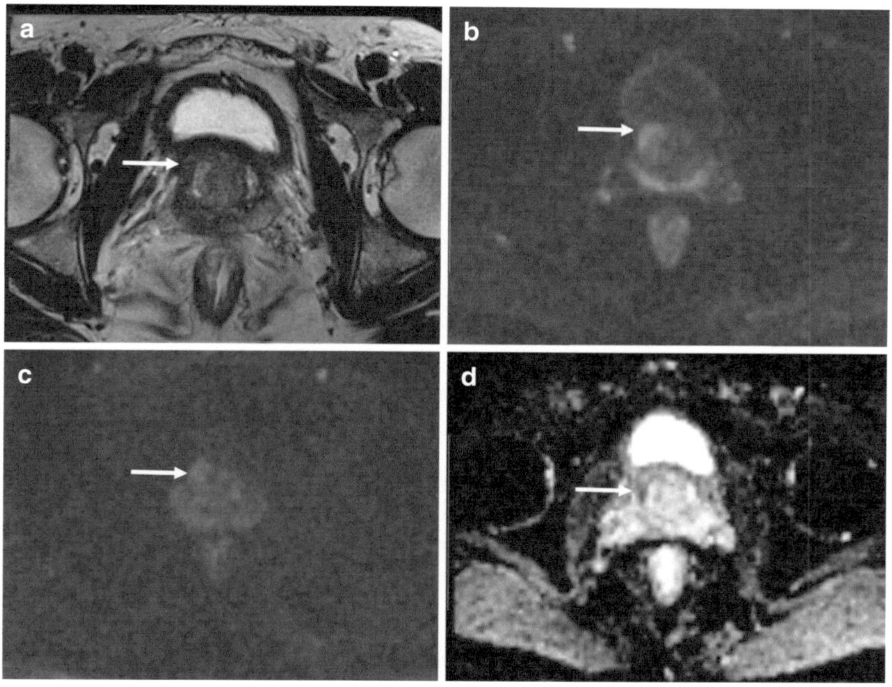

Fig. 6.3 Axial T2 weighted image shows a crescentic lesion at base of the prostate extending along the surgical capsule (**a**). There is marked diffusion restriction, denoted by the bright signal on high b-value 1000 s/mm^2 (**b**) and 1400 s/mm^2 (**c**) images and drop in signal on apparent diffusion coefficient (ADC) map (**d**). On targeted biopsy, this was reported as Gleason 7 prostate cancer

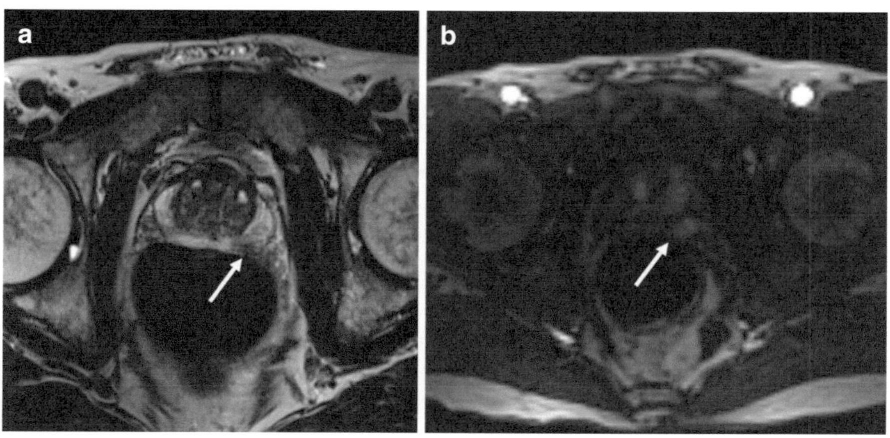

Fig. 6.4 Axial T2 weighted image (**a**) shows a ill-defined, diffuse lesion in left peripheral zone (**a**) with early enhancement on dynamic contrast enhanced image (**b**). On biopsy this was shown to be a low-grade cancer with Gleason score of 6

Locations Other Than Peripheral Zone

Anterior Fibromuscular Stroma The anterior fibromuscular stroma forms the anterior part of the prostate and is dark on T2 weighted images. *Cancers in this anterior location are often missed on standard biopsies. However, in a clinical scenario of multiple negative standard TRUS biopsies and rising PSA, MRI often identifies an anterior tumor in 8–20% of these patients* [7–9]. Anterior fibromuscular stroma cancers are typically lenticular shaped, show drop in diffusion coefficient and early contrast enhancement on DCE-MRI. DCE-MRI may actually facilitate the detection of tumor foci in anterior fibromuscular stroma since the normal anterior fibromuscular stroma is inherently hypovascular with persistent contrast enhancement while tumors show early enhancement and washout [5]. In addition, there may be a focal contour bulge in this location which is highly suspicious for tumor with extraprostatic extension (Figs. 6.5 and 6.6).

Central Zone The central zone is seen at the posterior base of the prostate surrounding the seminal vesicles and ejaculatory ducts. The normal central zone has low signal on T2 weighted images, is bilaterally symmetrical and extends up to the verumontanum, and is best seen in the coronal plane. The normal central zone also shows low

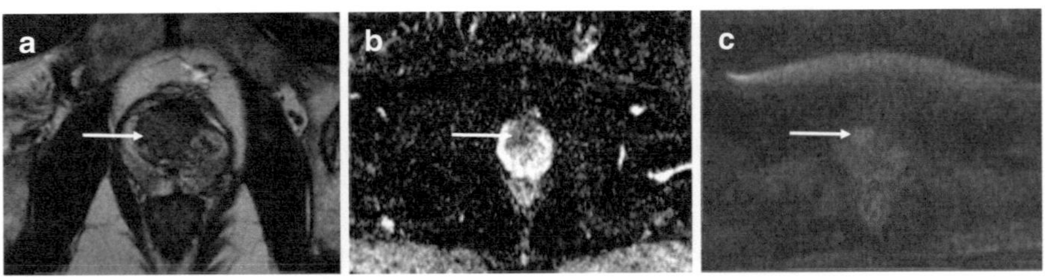

Fig. 6.5 Tumor within anterior fibromuscular stroma. Axial T2 weighted image shows a large lesion involving anterior transition zone and anterior fibromuscular stroma (**a**) with definite diffusion restriction (**b**, **c**). On biopsy this was Gleason 7 (4 + 3 = 7) prostate cancer

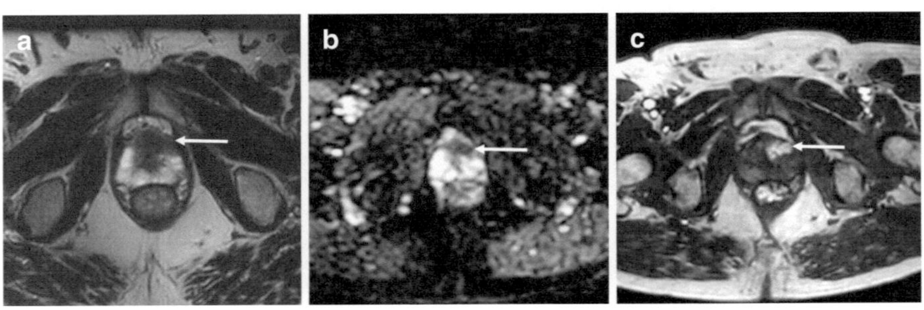

Fig. 6.6 Tumor within anterior fibromuscular stroma. Axial T2 weighted image (**a**) shows an asymmetrical looking anterior fibromuscular stroma with greater extension on to the left side. There is signal drop on apparent diffusion coefficient map (**b**). However the presence of focal early enhancement in the left half of the anterior fibromuscular stroma (arrow, **c**) is the most suspicious finding and the combination of these features greatly increases the probability of cancer being present (PI-RADS 5). On biopsy this was a Gleason 7 (4 + 3 = 7) prostate cancer

apparent diffusion coefficient due to its high stromal composition. In patients with benign prostatic hyperplasia (BPH), the enlarged transition zone distorts and compresses the central zone towards the base. In such cases, the central zone may not be seen distinctly from the transition zone and the normal central zone may be mistaken as a large transition zone nodule at base of prostate. This leads to over-scoring with PI-RADS and a false positive MRI read. More importantly, due to its low apparent diffusion coefficient and low signal on T2 weighted image, foci of cancer may be missed within the central zone. Clues to cancer within the central zone lie in the asymmetric appearance of central zone or presence of a focal lesion with even more pronounced dark signal on T2 weighted images and apparent diffusion coefficient maps as compared to the surrounding central zone. This focal abnormality may be corroborated with an early enhancement pattern on DCE-MRI (Fig. 6.7).

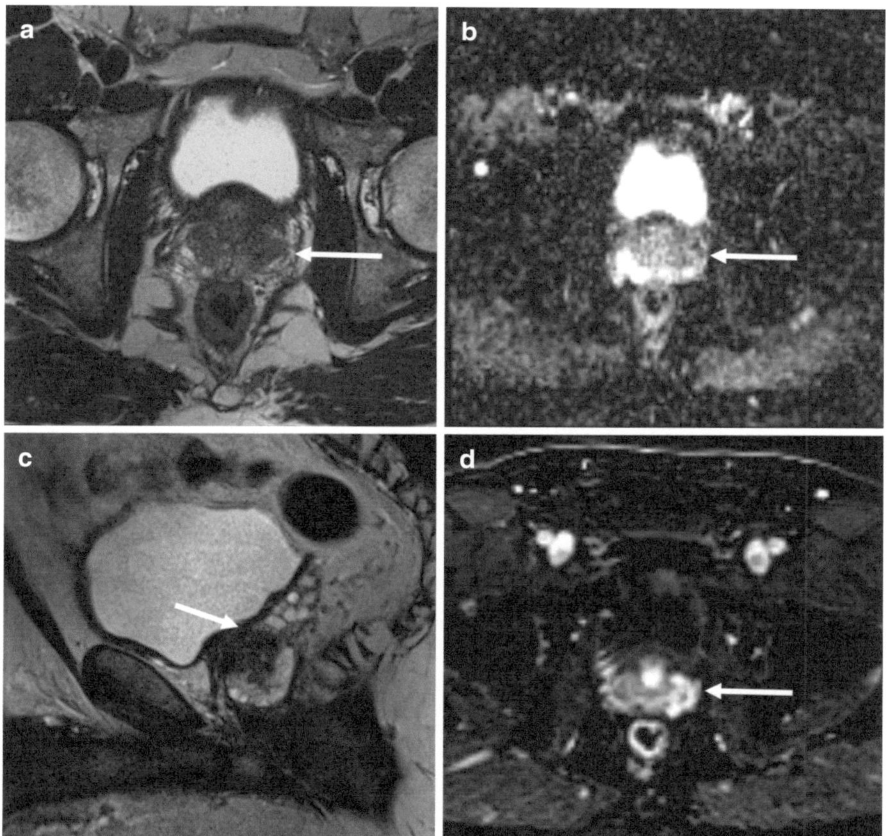

Fig. 6.7 Tumor in central zone. Axial T2 weighted image (**a**) at the cranial most aspect of the prostate base shows a focal dark lesion in left posteromedial peripheral zone (arrow, **a**) with mild signal drop on apparent diffusion coefficient map (arrow, **b**). On sagittal section (**c**), the abnormality is localized to the central zone of prostate (junction of posterior base and seminal vesicle). There is also focal early contrast enhancement (arrow, **d**). These findings upgrade overall score to PI-RADS 5 and targeted biopsy showed prostate cancer

Tumor Hidden Within Benign Hyperplastic Nodule Hyperplastic nodules are very heterogeneous in appearance and may obscure tumor foci. In addition, stromal hyperplastic nodules can mimic tumors due to low T2 weighted signal, low ADC and early contrast enhancement. Thus transition zone cancers are inherently harder to detect against a background of benign prostatic hyperplasia (BPH). However, looking for a uniform dark signal with indistinct margins (erased charcoal sign) within a BPH nodule is helpful [10]. Also, an ultra-high b-value DWI may show these tumor foci as bright areas against a background of suppressed signal from rest of the prostate [11, 12] (Figs. 6.8 and 6.9).

Periurethral Tumor The periurethral region, while pathologically being distinct from transition zone, is not seen separately on MRI. It is seen as a nonspecific area of decreased signal on T2 weighted image, which hampers visualization of tumor foci in this region. However, multiparametric MRI with diffusion weighted imaging and DCE-MRI may help in additional detection of periurethral tumors (Figs. 6.10 and 6.11).

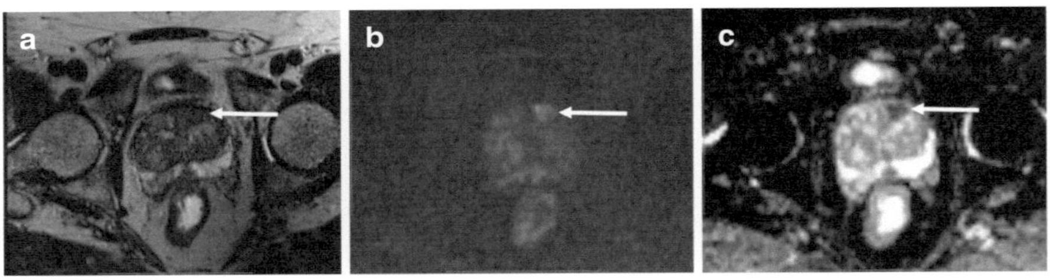

Fig. 6.8 Tumor against background of benign hyperplastic nodules. Axial T2 weighted image (**a**) shows enlarged transition zone with multiple hyperplastic nodules. Anteriorly is a focal nodule with low signal intensity (arrow, **a**) and marked diffusion restriction (**b**, **c**) suggestive of cancer

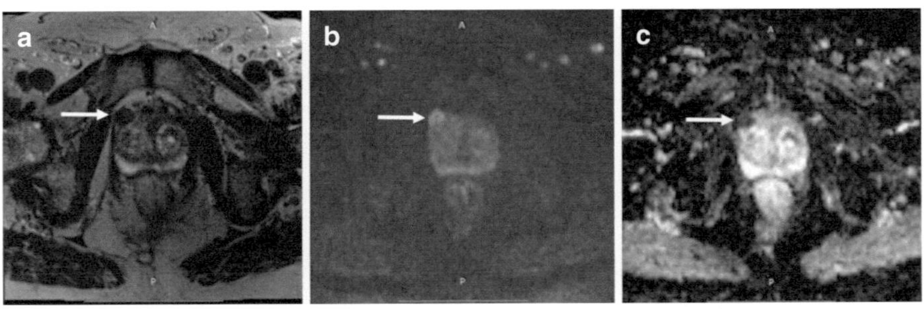

Fig. 6.9 Exophytic transition zone nodule with cancer. Axial T2 weighted image (**a**) shows enlarged transition zone with multiple hyperplastic nodules. Anteriorly is a focal exophytic nodule with low signal intensity (arrow, **a**) and marked diffusion restriction (**b**, **c**) and targeted biopsy showed cancer

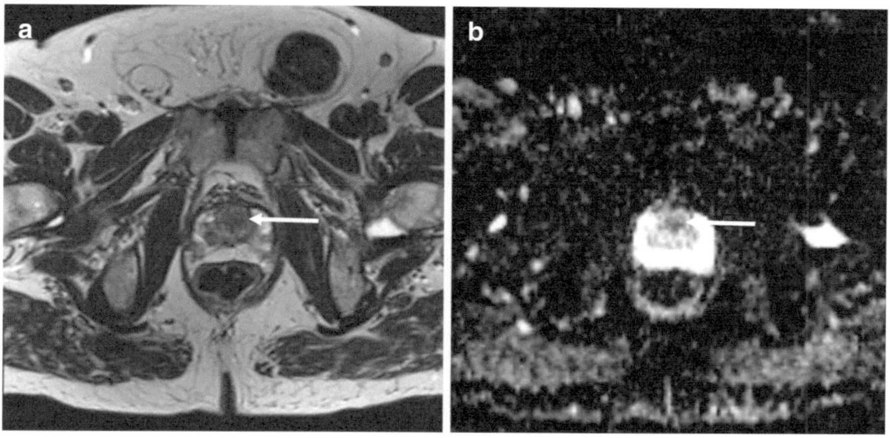

Fig. 6.10 Axial T2 weighted image of prostate apex shows a focal lesion in anterior periurethral region (arrow, **a**). The lesion can be hard to detect on T2 weighted image due to background dark signal in periurethral region. However the signal drop on apparent diffusion coefficient map (arrow, **b**) is suspicious and targeted biopsy showed Gleason 7 prostate cancer

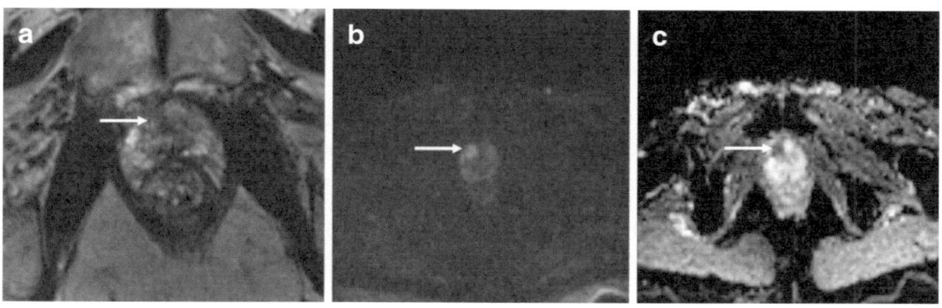

Fig. 6.11 Axial T2 weighted image of apical periurethral region prostate apex shows a small subtle lesion in anterior aspect (arrow, **a**). However there is marked diffusion restriction (**b**, **c**), which enables better detection of tumor

To summarize, cancers in anterior, apical and central zone of prostate are harder to detect on MRI. Relying predominantly on T2 weighted images for central zone and diffusion weighted imaging for apical peripheral zone tumors may lead to missing these atypical tumors. Hence it is worthwhile to visually assess all pulse sequences including DCE-MRI for all patients to improve the overall accuracy of multiparametric MRI in detecting prostate cancer.

References

1. Nix JW, Turkbey B, Hoang A, Volkin D, Yerram N, Chua C, et al. Very distal apical prostate tumours: identification on multiparametric MRI at 3 Tesla. BJU Int. 2012;110(11b):E694–700.
2. Iremashvili V, Pelaez L, Jorda M, Manoharan M, Arianayagam M, Rosenberg DL, et al. Prostate sampling by 12-core biopsy: comparison of the biopsy results with tumor location in prostatectomy specimens. Urology. 2012;79(1):37–42.
3. Kim JW, Park HK, Kim HG, Ham DY, Paick SH, Lho YS, et al. Discordance between location of positive cores in biopsy and location of positive surgical margin following radical prostatectomy. Korean J Urol. 2015;56(10):710–6.
4. Radtke JP, Boxler S, Kuru TH, Wolf MB, Alt CD, Popeneciu IV, et al. Improved detection of anterior fibromuscular stroma and transition zone prostate cancer using biparametric and multiparametric MRI with MRI-targeted biopsy and MRI-US fusion guidance. Prostate Cancer Prostatic Dis. 2015;18(3):288–96.
5. Rosenkrantz AB, Verma S, Turkbey B. Prostate cancer: top places where tumors hide on multiparametric MRI. Am J Roentgenol. 2015;204(4):W449–56.
6. Langer DL, van der Kwast TH, Evans AJ, Sun L, Yaffe MJ, Trachtenberg J, et al. Intermixed normal tissue within prostate cancer: effect on MR imaging measurements of apparent diffusion coefficient and T2—sparse versus dense cancers. Radiology. 2008;249(3):900–8.
7. Lawrentschuk N, Haider MA, Daljeet N, Evans A, Toi A, Finelli A, et al. "Prostatic evasive anterior tumours": the role of magnetic resonance imaging. BJU Int. 2010;105(9):1231–6.
8. Komai Y, Numao N, Yoshida S, Matsuoka Y, Nakanishi Y, Ishii C, et al. High diagnostic ability of multiparametric magnetic resonance imaging to detect anterior prostate cancer missed by transrectal 12-core biopsy. J Urol. 2013;190(3):867–73.
9. Hambrock T, Somford DM, Hoeks C, Bouwense SAW, Huisman H, Yakar D, et al. Magnetic resonance imaging guided prostate biopsy in men with repeat negative biopsies and increased prostate specific antigen. J Urol. 2010;183(2):520–7.
10. Akin O, Sala E, Moskowitz CS, Kuroiwa K, Ishill NM, Pucar D, et al. Transition zone prostate cancers: features, detection, localization, and staging at endorectal MR imaging. Radiology. 2006;239(3):784–92.
11. Jung SI, Donati OF, Vargas HA, Goldman D, Hricak H, Akin O. Transition zone prostate cancer: incremental value of diffusion-weighted endorectal MR imaging in tumor detection and assessment of aggressiveness. Radiology. 2013;269(2):493–503.
12. Hoeks CMA, Hambrock T, Yakar D, Hulsbergen-van de Kaa CA, Feuth T, Witjes JA, et al. Transition zone prostate cancer: detection and localization with 3-T multiparametric MR imaging. Radiology. 2013;266(1):207–17.

Tumor Mimics: Benign Conditions that Mimic Prostate Cancer

7

Ananya Panda and Vikas Gulani

The prostate gland is affected by a variety of other pathologies, apart from prostate cancer. While the main objective of multiparametric MRI is evaluation of prostate cancer, a variety of normal structures as well as benign pathologies can mimic prostate cancer. This chapter depicts the MR appearances of normal structures and benign pathologies that may be mistaken for prostate cancer.

Normal Structures that May Be Mistaken for Prostate Cancer

The reader is also referred to previous chapters (refer Normal Anatomy and Atypical Locations). Normal structures that can be mistaken for prostate cancer have been tabulated in Table 7.1 and depicted in subsequent figures (Figs. 7.1, 7.2, 7.3, 7.4, and 7.5).

Benign Conditions that May Be Mistaken for Prostate Cancer

Prostatitis: Prostatitis, either acute or chronic, can affect both the peripheral zone and the transition zone and comprises the most common cause of false-positive findings on MRI. A review of in-gantry biopsy specimens showed that more than half of targeted lesions were prostatitis on pathology [3, 4]. Chronic prostatitis is often subclincial and thus can be seen in MRIs of patients with elevated prostate specific antigen (PSA) without any prior history of prostatitis.

A. Panda
Department of Radiology, Mayo Clinic, Rochester, MN, USA
e-mail: panda.ananya@mayo.edu

V. Gulani (✉)
Fred Jenner Hodges Professor and Chair, Department of Radiology, University of Michigan, Ann Arbor, MI, USA
e-mail: vikasgulani@med.umich.edu

A. Panda et al. (eds.), *Reading MRI of the Prostate*,
https://doi.org/10.1007/978-3-319-99357-7_7

Table 7.1 Normal structures that may be mistaken for prostate cancer

	Normal structure	Reason for mimicking tumor	Clues to normal structure	Figures
1	Anterior Fibromuscular Stroma	Dark signal on T2 weighted image, low appparent diffusion coefficient (ADC) due to compact fibromuscular composition	• Midline, anterior location • Bilateral symmetrical, smooth outline • No focal bulge or irregularity in outline • Slow, persistent contrast enhancement	Fig. 7.1
2	Central zone	Dark on T2 weighted image, low ADC Loss of central zone-transition zone interface and compressed central zone secondary to BPH may cause central zone to be mistaken as tumor	• Typical location at posterior base of prostate • Bilateral symmetrical, conical configuration, best seen in coronal plane	Fig. 7.2
3	Thickened surgical capsule	Focally thickened surgical capsule shows low ADC and may be mistaken for tumor on DWI (especially if there is anatomic distortion on DWI)	• Knowledge of normal anatomy and location of surgical capsule between transition zone and peripheral zone • Correlation of low ADC structure with normal surgical capsule on T2 weighted image • Linear/band-like configuration	Fig. 7.3
4	Periprostatic veins	High signal on DWI, low ADC, partial volume effects and poorly defined prostate outlines at prostate apex may cause veins to be mistaken as tumor	• Location: Anterolateral to prostate • Tubular structures that can be tracked on consecutive images • Contrast enhancement confirms normal venous structures	Fig. 7.4
5	Periprostatic neurovascular bundle (NVB)	Normal nerves appear as signal void (dark) on ADC and have low signal intensity on T2 weighted image. These closely abut peripheral zone and hence may be mistaken for peripheral zone tumors, especially on ADC map and corresponding high b-value DWI due to anatomic distortion	• Location: 5 and 7 'o' clock positions posterolateral to prostate • Normal NVB can be tracked on consecutive images • Associated veins in NVB show contrast enhancement	Fig. 7.5

ADS apparent diffusion coefficient, *DWI* diffusion weighted imaging
Table references [1, 2]

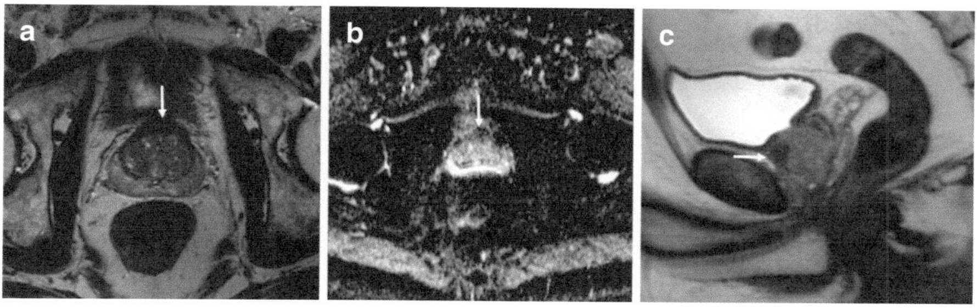

Fig. 7.1 Anterior Fibromuscular Stroma. The normal anterior stroma due to its dark signal on T2 weighted image (arrows, **a**, **c**) and signal drop on apparent diffusion coefficient map (arrow, **b**) can be mistaken for cancer

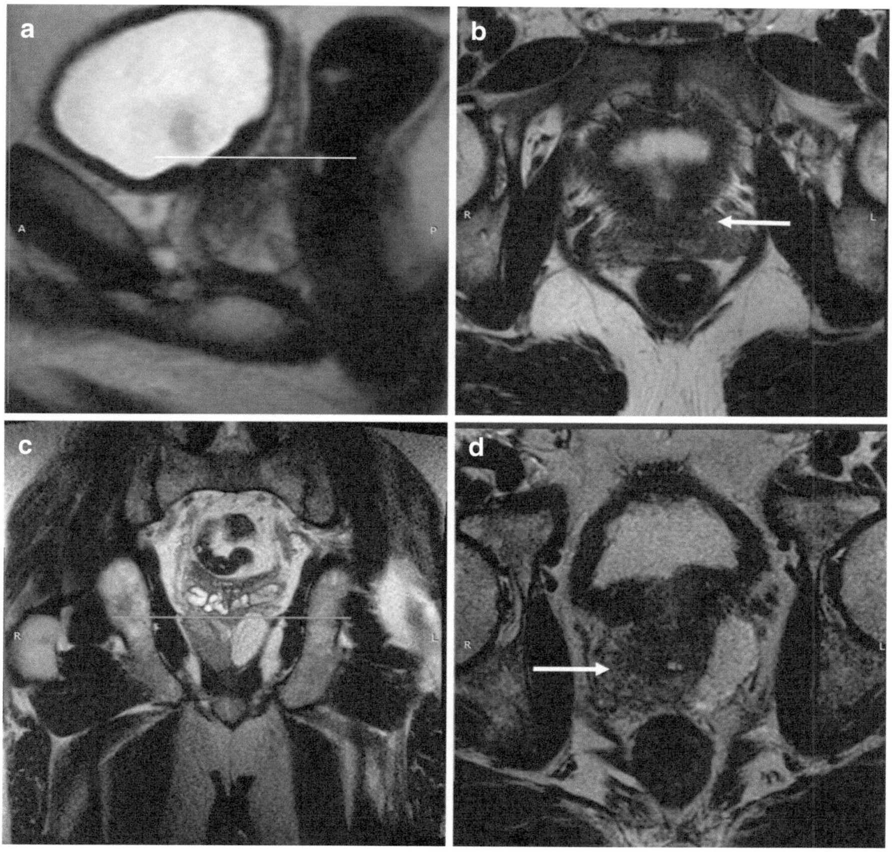

Fig. 7.2 Central gland. T2 weighted images from two different patients with transverse sections (**b**, **d**) obtained at the base of prostate cutting through the central gland (reference lines **a**, **c**) show the normal central gland in posteromedial base. When axial sections are viewed in isolation, central gland may be mistaken as a focal lesion, and viewing along with sagittal/coronal images can confirm the presence of normal central gland

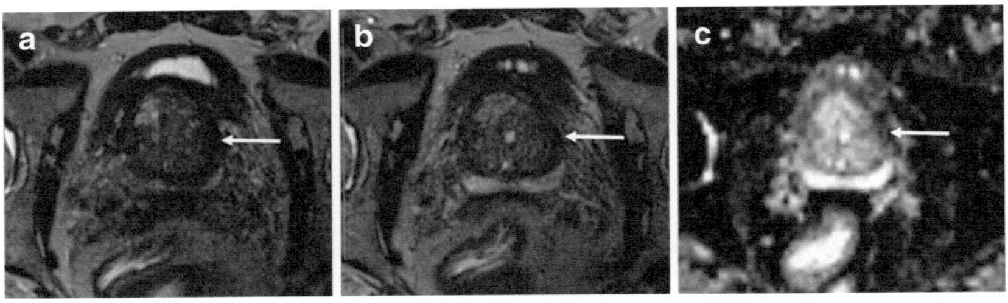

Fig. 7.3 Thickened surgical capsule. Focal thickening of the surgical capsule can be mistaken for a tumor due to dark signal on T2 weighted image (arrow **a**, **b**) and signal drop on apparent diffusion coefficient maps (arrow, **c**)

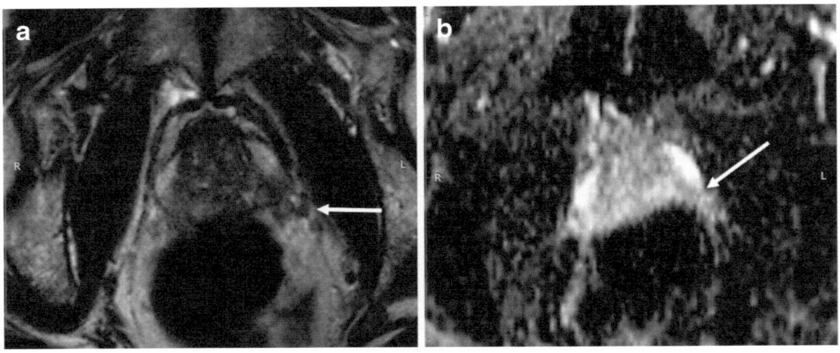

Fig. 7.4 MRI shows diffusion restriction at left posterolateral aspect at 5 'o' clock position (arrow, **b**), which may be mistaken as tumor. However on transverse T2 weighted image (**a**), this area corresponds to the location of periprostatic veins (arrow, **a**) which are closely related to the outer capsule of prostate

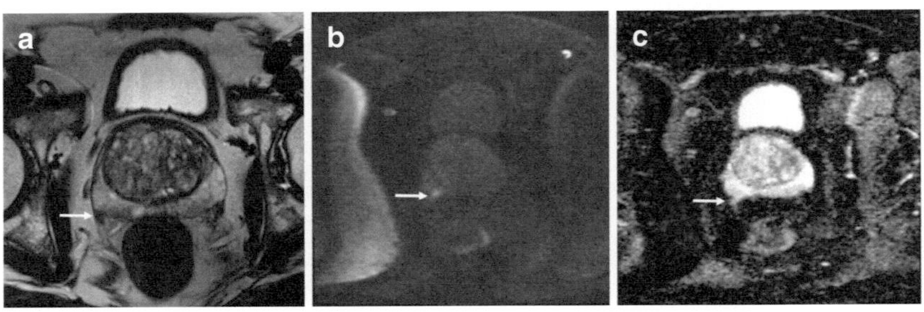

Fig. 7.5 Neurovascular bundles at typical 5 'o' clock and 7 'o' clock positions appear dark on T2 weighted images (arrow, **a**) and can show diffusion restriction, appearing bright on high b-value diffusion weighted image (arrow, **b**) with mild signal drop on corresponding apparent diffusion coefficient map (arrow, **c**)

Based on morphology, prostatitis may be partially separated from prostate cancer. Prostatitis is typically ill defined, linear or wedge-shaped in morphology without a definitive mass–like shape. Prostatitis also tends to be more diffusely distributed or may have a lobar distribution [5] (Fig. 7.6). However, prostatitis can *also* be

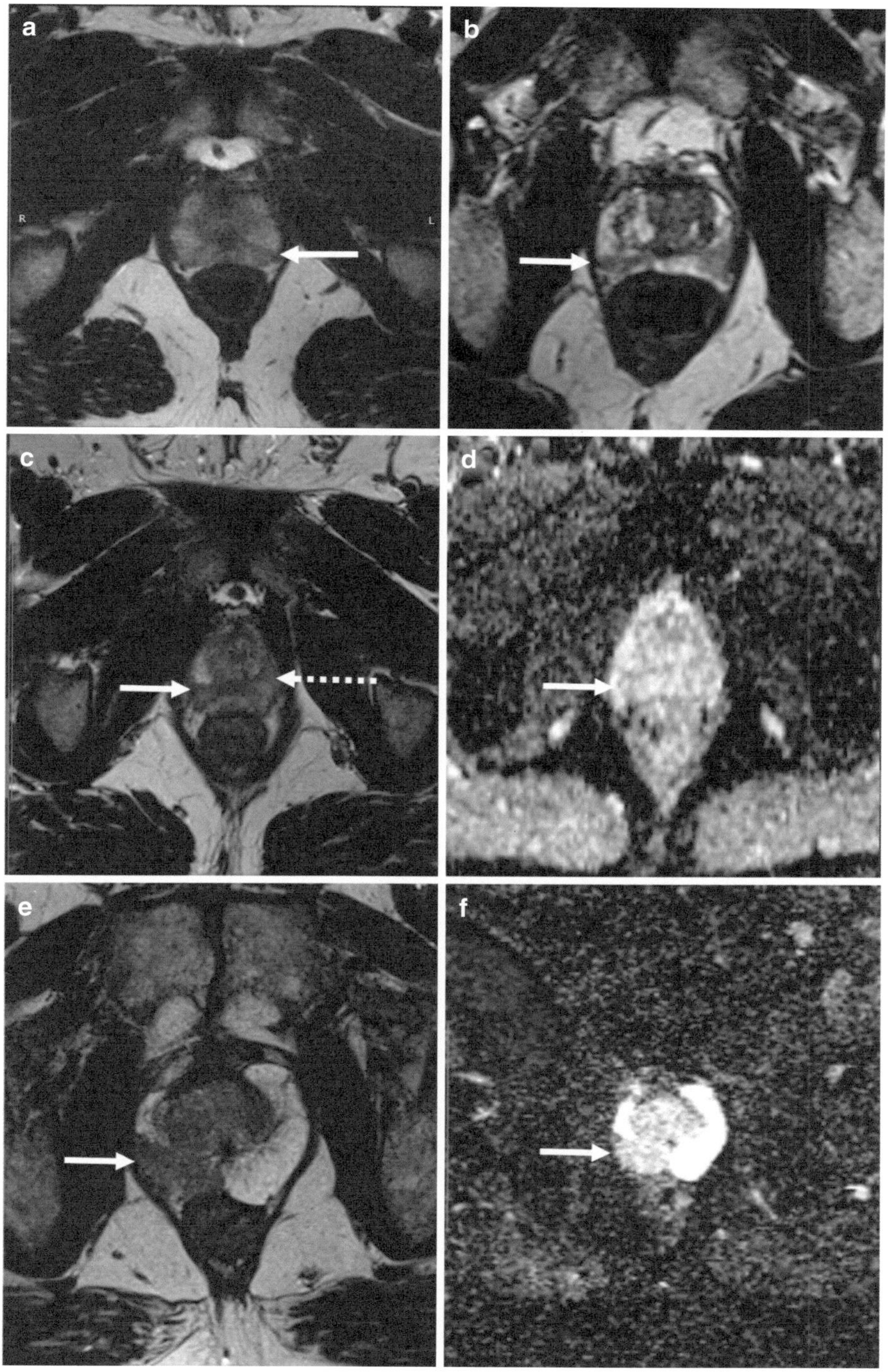

Fig. 7.6 Prostatitis in the Peripheral Zone. Lesions that are wedge-shaped with sharp borders (**a**, **b**), bilateral or diffuse (**c**) or have a lobar configuration (**e**) with mild signal drop on apparent diffusion coefficient maps (**d**, **f**) are likely to be prostatitis

focal, and focal prostatitis can be especially hard to differentiate from peripheral zone tumors. Diffusion weighted imaging and apparent diffusion coefficient mapping may help as prostatitis have a higher median apparent diffusion coefficient than prostate cancer [6]. Prostatitis in the transition zone can also mimic cancer by having the same "erased charcoal appearance" and low T2 weighted appearance as prostate cancer (Fig. 7.7).

Granulomatous prostatitis is a separate entity and can be either infective or inflammatory/immunologic in origin. Infective granulomatous prostatitis is most commonly caused by Mycobacterium tuberculosis either due to hematogeneous spread or direct

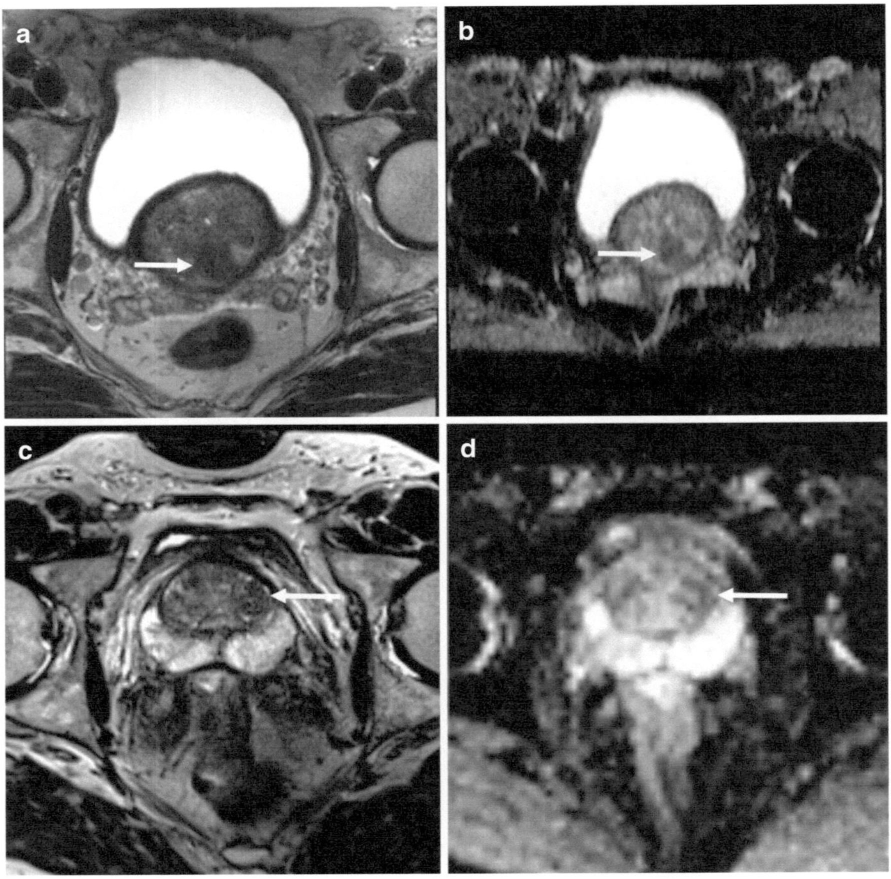

Fig. 7.7 Biopsy Proven cases of Prostatitis in Transition Zone. Axial T2 weighted image (**a**) shows a focal lesion with moderately low signal intensity and erased charcoal appearance (arrow, **a**) and signal drop on apparent diffusion coefficient map (arrow, **b**). The lesion was scored as PI-RADS 3 and biopsy showed prostatitis. Axial T2 weighted image (**a**) shows an oval lesion with well-defined borders and low signal intensity (arrow, **c**) and mild signal drop on apparent diffusion coefficient map (arrow, **d**). Again the lesion was coed as PI-RADS 3 and biopsy showed prostatitis

extension from adjacent organs. In the Western world, granulomatous prostatitis is often secondary to intravesical Bacillus-Calmette Guérin (BCG) therapy for urinary bladder cancer. Granulomatous prostatitis is clinically mistaken for cancer due to nodularity on digital rectal examination and elevated PSA. On MRI, it also has a focal morphology and appearances similar to that of prostate cancer [7, 8] (Fig. 7.8). Hence differentiation can be difficult unless there is a specific known history of tuberculosis infection or BCG therapy. One helpful feature described for this condition is presence of early and prolonged rim contrast enhancement [9].

Atrophy is pathologically characterized by glandular crowding due to volume loss. It can be secondary to inflammation, treatment, biopsy or ischemia. Due to glandular and nuclear crowding, it appears dark on T2 weighted images and has low

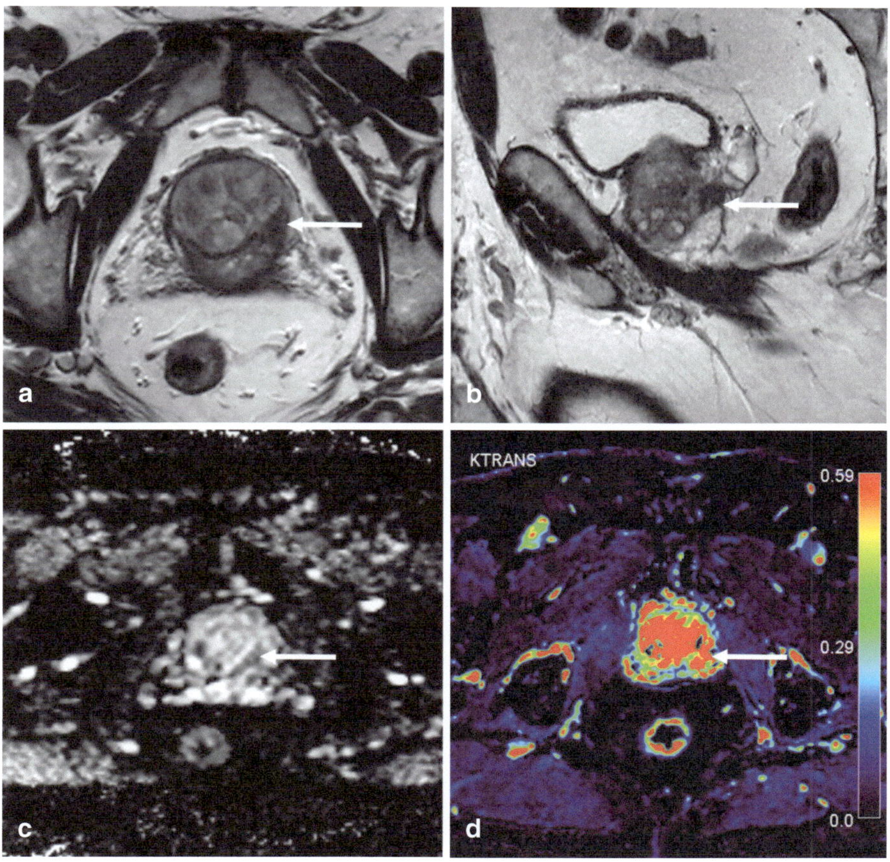

Fig. 7.8 Biopsy proven case of granulomatous prostatitis. T2 weighted images show a lesion with low signal intensity in left base peripheral zone (arrow, **a**) also extending up to seminal vesicle (**b**) The lesion has signal drop on the apparent diffusion coefficient map (**c**) and shows early enhancement and increased perfusion (arrow, **d**). These appearances are highly suggestive of malignancy, however biopsy showed non-mycobacterial granulomatous prostatitis

apparent diffusion coefficient values. In addition, the glandular damage in atrophy releases PSA into blood, leading to elevated serum PSA [10]. Thus focal atrophy comprises another false-positive finding on MRI (Fig. 7.9). If the atrophy involves a larger area, it is usually associated with volume loss and this can help differentiate it from cancers (Fig. 7.10).

Stromal hyperplastic nodule in Transition Zone: In BPH, the transition zone has a markedly heterogeneous appearance, due to a combination of glandular and stromal hyperplasia. While glandular hyperplasia is easy to identify due to increased signal on T2 weighted images, stromal hyperplasia can be hard to differentiate from prostate cancer. Stromal hyperplasia is dark on T2 weighted images, shows low

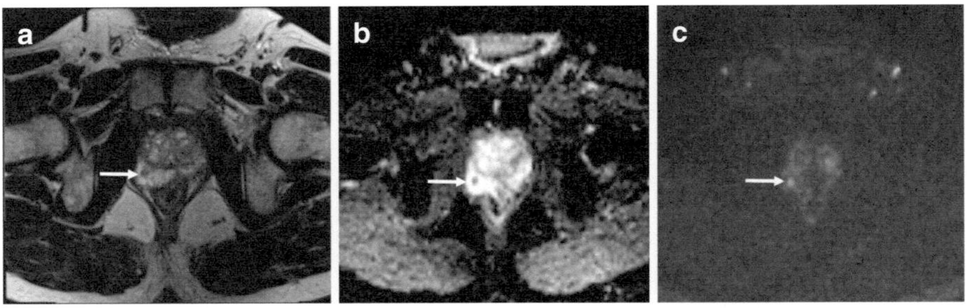

Fig. 7.9 Biopsy proven case of atrophy. Axial T2 weighted image (**a**) showed a small well-defined focal lesion in right peripheral zone (arrow, **a**) with definite diffusion restriction (**b**, **c**). The lesion was scored as PI-RADS 4 and targeted biopsy was performed which showed focal atrophy and no evidence of malignancy

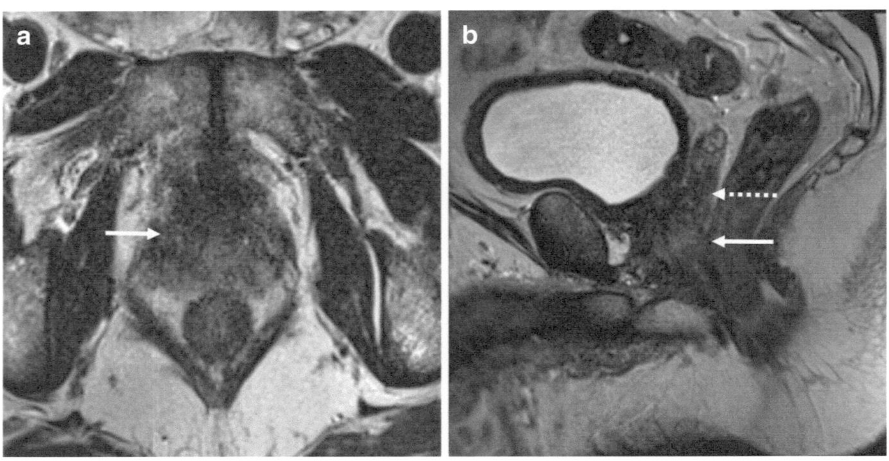

Fig. 7.10 Post-radiation atrophy. T2 weighted images of a patient who previously underwent radiation therapy show that that the prostate has diffuse dark signal with irregular capsular outline (arrow, **a**). The seminal vesicle also shows low signal (dotted arrow, **b**) with loss of rectoprostatic fat plane (arrow, **b**). These appearances can be mistaken for cancer if previous history of radiation therapy is not known

apparent diffusion coefficient and early enhancement on DCE-MRI, similar to prostate cancer [11]. Based on shape and morphology of lesion, it may partially be possible to differentiate stromal BPH nodule from transition zone cancer. Stromal BPH nodules are generally round or spherical in shape, with discrete, encapsulated margins. On the other hand, lenticular/teardrop shape, irregular margins and local invasion are suggestive of transition zone tumor [12, 13]. Despite these morphological differences, it is hard to distinguish the two entities and diagnosis can be confirmed only by targeted biopsy (Figs. 7.11 and 7.12).

Occasionally a transition zone nodule may extrude into the peripheral zone and may be inadvertently mistaken for a peripheral zone tumor due to low signal on T2 weighted image and low apparent diffusion coefficient. However, the well-circumscribed, encapsulated margins and continuity of the lesion with transition zone confirms its benign nature.

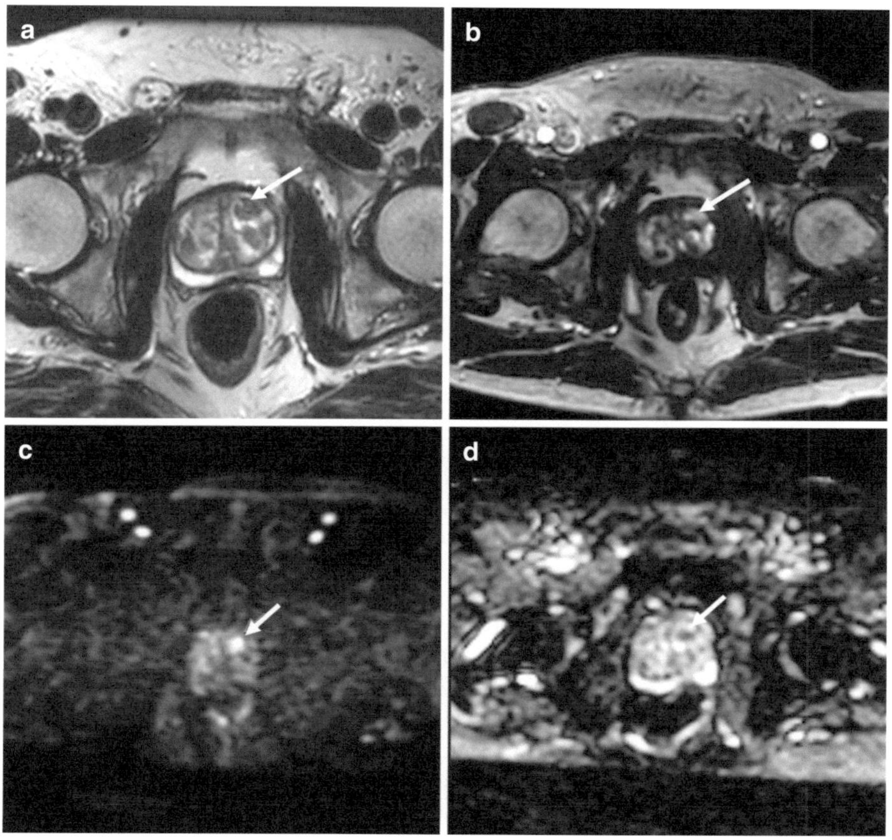

Fig. 7.11 Biopsy proven case of stromal hyperplasia. T2 weighted axial image shows a lenticular lesion in left anterior transition zone (arrow, A) with early contrast enhancement (arrow, **b**). The lesion is also bright on high b-value diffusion weighted image (arrow, **c**) with signal drop on corresponding apparent diffusion coefficient map (arrow, **d**). These findings are highly suspicious of malignancy, however targeted biopsy showed stromal hyperplasia

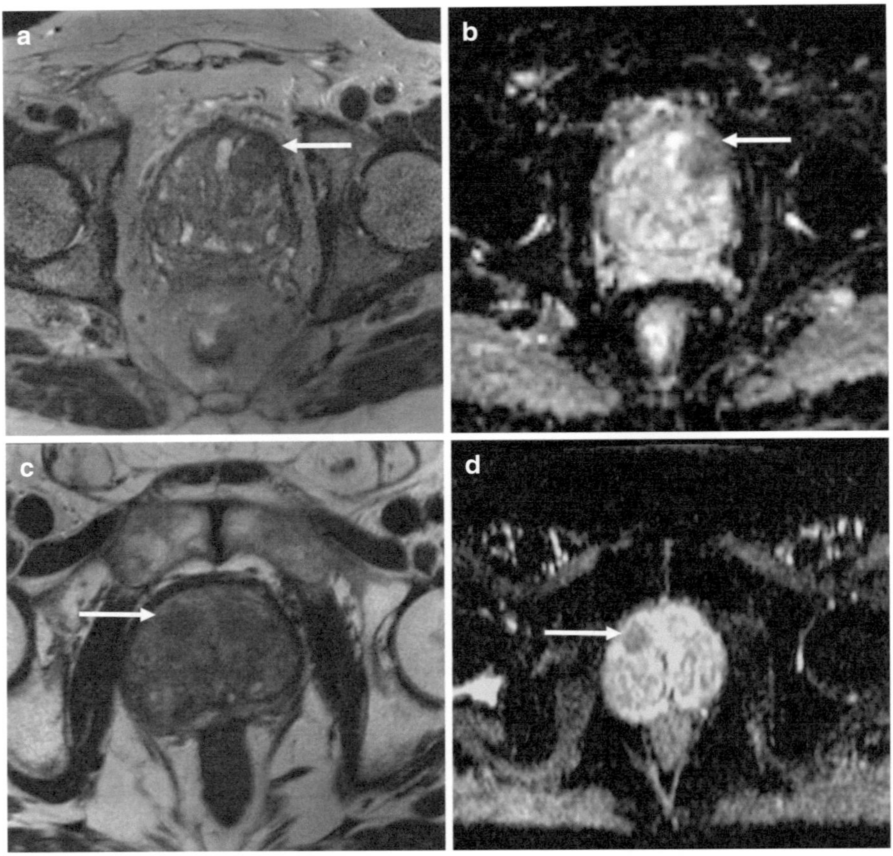

Fig. 7.12 Biopsy proven cases of stromal hyperplasia. T2 weighted axial images from two different patients show transition zone hypertrophy with well-defined nodules with moderately low signal intensity in anterior transition zone (arrows **a**, **c**). Both lesions show signal drop on apparent diffusion coefficient maps (arrows **b**, **d**). Targeted biopsy for both lesions showed benign prostatic tissue with stromal hyperplasia

Post-biopsy hemorrhage: Hemorrhage after prostate biopsy occurs more commonly in peripheral zone than in transition zone and the imaging sequelae can persist for several weeks. Hemorrhage can be confused with tumor due to its low signal intensity on T2 weighted images and dark appearance on apparent diffusion coefficient maps. However, on correlation with other sequences, hemorrhage is bright on T1 weighted images and does not have bright signal on high b-value images. Thus it can be differentiated from tumors. In addition, the "hemorrhage exclusion" sign in which hemorrhage is seen to outline the tumor on T1w image can help in detecting underlying tumors [14].

Calcifications: Prostatic calcifications are commonly seen with aging and represent dystrophic calcifications in the glands. Calcifications typically occur in the transition zone. They appear intensely dark on all sequences since they represent

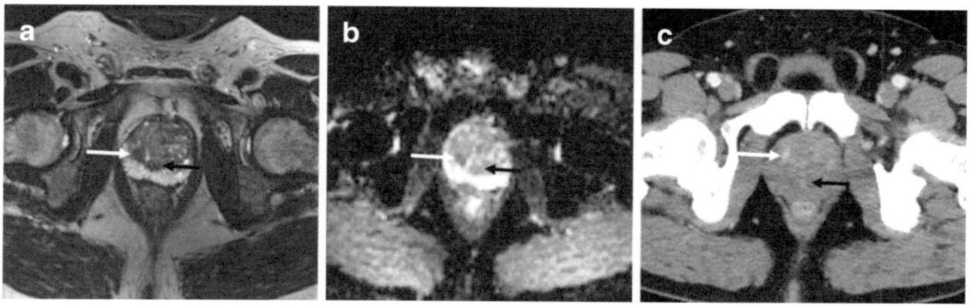

Fig. 7.13 Prostatic calcifications. Axial T2 weighted image (**a**) shows two focal lesions in posterior transition zone with low signal intensity (arrows, **a**) and signal drop on apparent diffusion coefficient maps (arrows, **b**). However corresponding CT scan shows presence of calcifications in same locations (arrows, **c**)

signal voids. While they may be mistaken for transition zone tumors on T2 weighted images, the dark appearance on all other sequences is a clue to presence of calcifications. In addition, correlation with CT scans if available, can confirm the presence of calcifications (Fig. 7.13).

References

1. Kitzing YX, Prando A, Varol C, Karczmar GS, Maclean F, Oto A. Benign conditions that mimic prostate carcinoma: MR imaging features with histopathologic correlation. Radiographics. 2015;36(1):162–75.
2. Rosenkrantz AB, Taneja SS. Radiologist, be aware: ten pitfalls that confound the interpretation of multiparametric prostate MRI. Am J Roentgenol. 2013;202(1):109–20.
3. Hambrock T, Fütterer JJ, Huisman HJ, Hulsbergen-vandeKaa C, van Basten J-P, van Oort I, et al. Thirty-two-channel coil 3T magnetic resonance-guided biopsies of prostate tumor suspicious regions identified on multimodality 3T magnetic resonance imaging: technique and feasibility. Investig Radiol. 2008;43(10):686–94.
4. Watanabe Y, Nagayama M, Araki T, Terai A, Okumura A, Amoh Y, et al. Targeted biopsy based on ADC map in the detection and localization of prostate cancer: a feasibility study. J Magn Reson Imaging JMRI. 2013;37(5):1168–77.
5. Shukla-Dave A, Hricak H, Eberhardt SC, Olgac S, Muruganandham M, Scardino PT, et al. Chronic prostatitis: MR imaging and 1H MR spectroscopic imaging findings--initial observations. Radiology. 2004;231(3):717–24.
6. Nagel KNA, Schouten MG, Hambrock T, Litjens GJS, Hoeks CMA, ten Haken B, et al. Differentiation of prostatitis and prostate cancer by using diffusion-weighted MR imaging and MR-guided biopsy at 3 T. Radiology. 2013;267(1):164–72.
7. Rais-Bahrami S, Nix JW, Turkbey B, Pietryga JA, Sanyal R, Thomas JV, et al. Clinical and multiparametric MRI signatures of granulomatous prostatitis. Abdom Radiol N Y. 2017;42(7):1956–62.
8. Gottlieb J, Princenthal R, Cohen MI. Multi-parametric MRI findings of granulomatous prostatitis developing after intravesical bacillus calmette-guérin therapy. Abdom Radiol N Y. 2017;42(7):1963–7.
9. Kawada H, Kanematsu M, Goshima S, Kondo H, Watanabe H, Noda Y, et al. Multiphase contrast-enhanced magnetic resonance imaging features of Bacillus Calmette-Guérin-induced granulomatous prostatitis in five patients. Korean J Radiol. 2015;16(2):342–8.

10. Prando A, Billis A. Focal prostatic atrophy: mimicry of prostatic cancer on TRUS and 3D-MRSI studies. Abdom Imaging. 2009;34(2):271–5.
11. Oto A, Kayhan A, Jiang Y, Tretiakova M, Yang C, Antic T, et al. Prostate cancer: differentiation of central gland cancer from benign prostatic hyperplasia by using diffusion-weighted and dynamic contrast-enhanced MR imaging. Radiology. 2010;257(3):715–23.
12. Akin O, Sala E, Moskowitz CS, Kuroiwa K, Ishill NM, Pucar D, et al. Transition zone prostate cancers: features, detection, localization, and staging at endorectal MR imaging. Radiology. 2006;239(3):784–92.
13. Hoeks CMA, Hambrock T, Yakar D, van de Kaa H–, CA FT, Witjes JA, et al. Transition zone prostate cancer: detection and localization with 3-T multiparametric MR imaging. Radiology. 2013;266(1):207–17.
14. Tamada T, Sone T, Jo Y, Yamamoto A, Yamashita T, Egashira N, et al. Prostate cancer: relationships between postbiopsy hemorrhage and tumor detectability at MR diagnosis. Radiology. 2008;248(2):531–9.

8 The Value of Incorporating Multiparametric MRI for Active Surveillance in Patients with Prostate Cancer

Amr Mahran, Kirtishri Mishra, Christina Buzzy, and Lee Ponsky

Active surveillance (AS) is an increasingly utilized treatment strategy for patients with low-risk prostate cancer consisting of careful, periodic monitoring with periodic PSA checks, digital rectal examination (DRE), and prostate biopsy with the intent to defer definitive treatment. This treatment strategy evolved to reduce overtreatment in men with indolent prostate cancer (PCa) without compromising oncological outcomes [1]. In low-risk PCa patients, AS has been evaluated and performs comparably to definitive modalities of treatment [2]. The American Urological Association (AUA) and the National Comperhensive Cancer Network (NCCN) recommended the utilization of AS in patients with very-low and low-risk disease (Table 8.1). In addition, AS may be considered a reasonable option for patients with favorable intermediate-risk disease; however, there is concern for the incidence of metastasis in these patients when compared to definitive treatment approaches [3, 4]. Multiparametric Magnetic Reasonance Imaging (mpMRI) of the prostate could be valuable in confirming the patients' candidacy for active surveillance and further monitoring of their disease progression.

The credibility of AS with long-term follow-up has been demonstrated in multiple prospective studies, indicating reasonable intervention-free rates and maintenance of a high health-related quality of life [5–7]. Men with low-risk disease on AS

A. Mahran · K. Mishra · C. Buzzy
Urology Institute, University Hospitals Cleveland Medical Center, Cleveland, OH, USA

Case Western Reserve University School of Medicine, Cleveland, OH, USA
e-mail: amr.mahran@uhhospitals.org; Kirtishri.Mishra2@UHhospitals.org; christina.antonopoulos@case.edu

L. Ponsky (✉)
Professor and Chair, Urology Institute, Leo and Charlotte Goldberg
Chair of Advanced Surgical Therapies, Master Clinician in Urologic Oncology, University Hospitals Cleveland Medical Center, Case Western Reserve University School of Medicine, Cleveland, OH, USA
e-mail: Lee.Ponsky@UHhospitals.org

A. Panda et al. (eds.), *Reading MRI of the Prostate*,
https://doi.org/10.1007/978-3-319-99357-7_8

Table 8.1 Eligibility of patients with organ-confined prostate cancer for AS

Risk group	Grade of recommendation	Level of evidence	Criteria
Very low-risk	Strong	Grade A	PSA <10 ng/ml AND Grade Group 1 "GS 3 + 3" AND clinical stage T1-T2a AND <34% of biopsy cores positive AND no core with >50% involved, AND PSA density <0.15 ng/ml/cc
Low-risk	Moderate	Grade B	PSA <10 ng/ml AND Grade Group 1 "GS 3 + 3" AND clinical stage T1-T2a
Intermediate risk (favorable)	Conditional	Grade C	Grade Group 1 "GS 3 + 3" (with PSA 10–<20) OR Grade Group 2 "GS 3 + 4" (with PSA<10)

have shown less than 3% prostate cancer–specific mortality at 10 years [2]. However, even with adherence to strict AS inclusion criteria, histopathological upgrading has been reported to occur in up to 28% of patients [8].

Current Standard of Care (SOC) for Active Surveillance

Patients on AS are currently monitored by three parameters including serum prostate specific antigen (PSA), digital rectal examination (DRE), and repeat prostate biopsy. Total PSA (protein bound and free, non-protein bound) should be performed every three to six months with the option of assessing free PSA at the discretion of the urologist. Total PSA doubling time <3 years or a total PSA increase >10–15 ng/mL are indications for a repeat transrectal ultrasound (TRUS)-guided biopsy. Yearly DRE is recommended to detect any palpable prostate lesions. A repeat prostate biopsy is generally accepted within the first year to rule out high grade disease that may have been missed on the original biopsy [9]. These tools are measures for assessing disease burden; however, even in combination, they may not always detect the extent of disease nor foresee the incidence of progression [10, 11].

Challenges with the Current SOC for AS and the Utility of Prostate MRI

Under-Sampling of the Prostate with TRUS-Guided Biopsy

About 40–60% of patients with at least one prior negative systematic biopsy may harbor undetected cancer [12]. The TRUS-guided biopsy method typically consists of two biopsy cores taken from six regions of the posterior peripheral zone for a total of 12 predetermined, systematically acquired cores. This is a "blind" procedure that depends on the regional sampling of the urologist performing the biopsy. The TRUS-guided biopsy technique can miss lesions located in the transition zone or in the anterior portion of the prostate and can underestimate cancerous lesion size located in the posterior peripheral zone [13]. Large multi-centered clinical trials have shown the increased accuracy of MRI over TRUS biopsy for detection of clinically significant disease. The PROMIS trial demonstrated the enhanced negative predictive value (NPV) of prostate multiparametric MRI (mpMRI) compared to TRUS-guided biopsy using transperineal mapping prostate biopsy as the reference test (89% versus 76% for Gleason Score (GS) $\geq 4 + 3$ PCa disease and 76% vs 63% for GS $\geq 3 + 4$ disease, respectively). Utilization of mpMRI resulted in upwards of 18% increased detection of clinically significant cancer when compared to the standard of care TRUS biopsy alone [14]. The PRECISION randomized-trial showed the superiority of MRI with or without targeted biopsy compared to standard TRUS biopsy with fewer men in the MRI-targeted biopsy group receiving a diagnosis of clinically insignificant disease compared to the standard-biopsy group [15].

Prostate MRI permits the localization of tumors and targeted biopsy guidance, which was not previously available. A large prospective study compared systematic biopsy, MRI- fusion biopsy, and combined techniques. It is evident that MRI targeting allows detection of more clinically significant cancers compared to systematic sampling alone [16]. MRI is able to identify almost 80% of prostate cancer lesions, however, the majority of PSA-detected cancers are not visualized on TRUS [17, 18]. mpMRI is specifically useful in detection of prostate cancer at challenging locations such as the anterior portion of the prostate, the transitional and central zones, and distal apical region [19] (Fig. 8.1). The American Urological Association has recently recommended MRI-guided biopsy in cases requiring a repeat biopsy [20].

Almost 20–30% of patients who were initially selected for active surveillance are offered curative-intent treatments such as surgery or radiation due to reclassification after targeting de-novo lesions identified on MRI [21, 22]. In one study, 51 out of 470 patients, initially included on active surveillance, had undergone

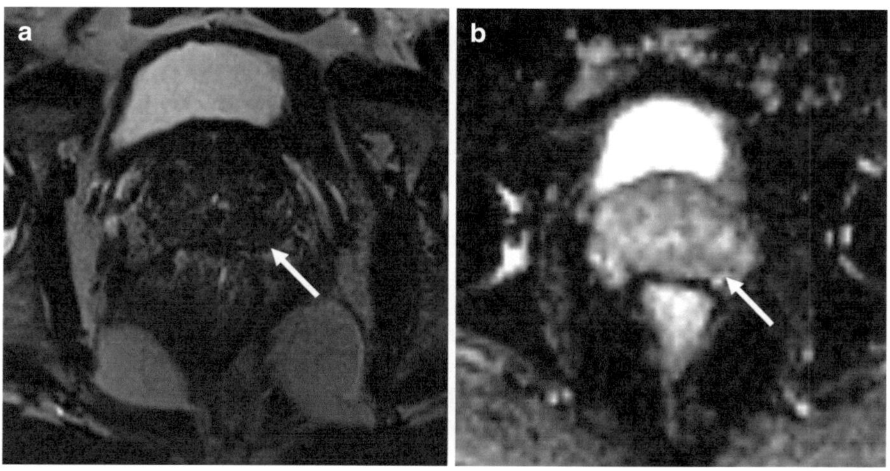

Fig. 8.1 Repeat in-gantry targeted biopsy of central gland lesion. Previous TRUS biopsy revealed low-grade prostate cancer (Gleason score $3 + 3 = 6$, 8% core involvement) from left base, other cores were negative and patient was kept on active surveillance. A follow-up MRI 1 year later showed ill-defined lesion in central gland (arrow, **a**) with low apparent diffusion coefficient (arrow, **b**) that was targeted with in-gantry biopsy. Repeat biopsy showed clinically significant prostate cancer (Gleason score $3 + 4 = 7$, core: 80% involvement)

radical prostatectomy after evidence of progression on repeat biopsy. In 75% of this subset of patients, progression occurred within 1–2 years after initial diagnosis which may infer missing the higher grade cancer on the initial biopsy rather than depicting actual cancer progression [9, 23].

MRI together with clinical data allows the identification and eligibility of patients for active surveillance [24]. Visible tumors on MRI are found to be associated with a Gleason score pathology that might make the patients no longer AS candidates, whereas a negative MRI was associated with a decreased risk of adverse biopsy pathology [25]. A recent meta-analysis reported that the risk of Gleason score upgrading increased from 27 to 43% after radical prostatectomy when there was a visible lesion on prostatic MRI [21]. Overall, the advantages of targeting MRI-visible lesions before AS enrollment include reducing the occurrence of sampling error, improving the assessment of the whole-prostate pathology, and eventually providing more positive cores and longer core lengths than traditional biopsy (Fig. 8.2). The continuous growth of MRI-guided biopsies is expected to improve the patients' criteria for AS enrollment [18, 26].

Necessity for Repeat Biopsy

Patients on AS require repeat biopsy along with regular PSA checks and DRE. As an invasive procedure, this makes these patients at increased risk of the undesired morbidities e.g. urinary retention, urinary tract infection, bacteremia, and possibly sepsis. Biopsy may be accompanied by other adverse events such as hematospermia (1.1–93%), hematuria >1 day (10–80%), rectal bleeding (1.3–45%), and prostatitis (1%) [27–32]. Hematuria lasting >3 days was reported in 22.6% of patients in a randomized study and was attributed with increased prostate and transition zone volumes. Others reported increased bleeding with more sampling of the prostate or larger needle size [32–35]. The number of cores was also associated with increased risk of rectal bleeding and hematospermia [36–38].

Another study showed that men on AS have a 30% increased odds of having associated infection with every prior biopsy, contributing to the increased incidence of multi-drug resistance and the financial burden of hospitalization due to infections associated with the TRUS biopsy procedure. They found that the number of previous biopsies was predictive of infectious complications [39]. Due to the emergence of fluoroquinolone resistance, about 2.3–3.6% of patients are hospitalized in England because of infections post- systematic biopsy adding great burden to the health system [40].

The negative predictive value of mpMRI varies throughout the literature, reaching greater than 95% for clinically significant cancer [41–43]. Patients with negative mpMRI are more suitable for AS compared to those with a detected tumor on mpMRI [43]. It is believed that a negative mpMRI in patients with very low-risk disease may be adequate to avoid repeat follow-up biopsies and consequently, the undesired complications associated with biopsy.

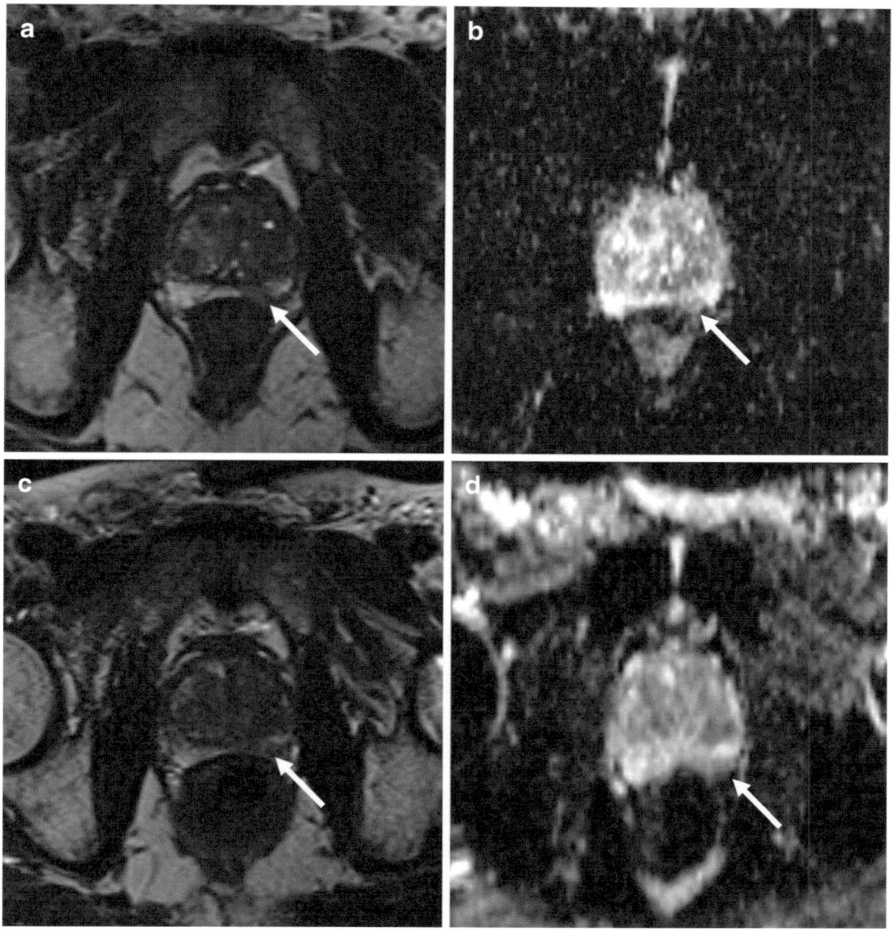

Fig. 8.2 Active Surveillance combined with Targeted Biopsy. Initial MRI for the patient (**a**, **b**) showed an ill-defined lesion in left peripheral zone (arrow) that was categorized as PI-RADS 3 lesion. The patient was kept on active surveillance. Follow-up MRI after 10 months (**c**, **d**) showed unchanged appearance of left peripheral zone lesion (arrow). On follow-up in-gantry targeted biopsy of the lesion was done was done which revealed low-grade/ Gleason score six cancer and patient continues to be on active surveillance

Non-tracking Systematic Biopsy in Active Surveillance

The conventional TRUS biopsy is a standard technique with systematically obtaining 12 cores from the apical, mid, and basal regions of the prostate. This random nature does not allow a trackable location of positive lesions on repeat biopsies. MRI-guided biopsy provided the advantage of tracking the location of biopsy cored whether within or away from the MRI-detected lesions. This advantage allows subsequent re-biopsy of the same location with anticipated accuracy within few millimeters [44]. In a study by Chang et al., patients who were selected for active surveillance after MRI/US fusion biopsies were followed for 1 year and then underwent a repeat MRI/US fusion biopsy using the tracking technology and non-tracking biopsy. 48 out of 91 (53%) patients diagnosed with Gleason upgrading were only identified by tracking (resampling of the previous positive spots) [45]. These upgraded patients would have been missed in case of using the non-tracking biopsy. This highlights the superiority of MRI-targeted biopsy given the accuracy of detection of patients who are no longer qualified for AS.

Biopsy Reclassification on Active Surveillance

Even with strict inclusion criteria, biopsy reclassification can occur within 9–40.5% of patients on AS [46, 47]. Reclassification was defined as either Gleason score upgrading, increased tumor volume, or both. Reasons for reclassifiation can be due either to natural disease progression or to having missed the higher-grade lesion on initial TRUS biopsy. Biopsy reclassification is the most critical factor for switching to definitive treatment in patients on AS. Eineluoto et al. reported that 74% of patients had intervention due to disease reclassification on biopsy [48]. Examining a cohort of 76 patients on AS for PCa with at least two consecutive prostate mpMRIs, they found that initial mpMRI PI-RADS 4 and 5 lesions were significantly associated with GS upgrading ($p = 0.008$) and treatment change ($p = 0.009$). They reported that about 69% of patients with GS progression on repeat mpMRI were significantly associated with changes in treatment decision. PI-RADS 4 and 5 index lesion demonstrated an average sensitivity of 80% and NPV of 93% when correlated with Gleason score upgrading [48].

In another study, authors retrospectively evaluated radical prostatectomy patients who were eligible for AS and had undergone preoperative 3 T mpMRI. They identified 263 (88.3%) patients with visible lesion on mpMRI. Almost 50% of those patients experienced Gleason score upgrading versus 14.3% of patients without MRI-visible lesions ($p < 0.001$). Also, 52.1% were diagnosed with unfavorable disease versus 14.3% of patients with non-detected cancer on MRI [49].

Anxiety

In a study performed by Tan et al., 15% and 14% of AS patients experienced significant anxiety either general anxiety or prostate specific anxiety, respectively [50]. Anderson et al. suggested a short trait-anxiety screening to help identify patients with clinically relevant anxiety and those at risk of reduced health related quality of life (HRQL) [51]. This anxiety could be in part due to the patient knowledge of prostate under-sampling on the initial biopsy. Having a negative mpMRI in addition to eligible Gleason score might help assure these patients and help reduce their anxiety. Another important point, if negative mpMRI replaces confirmatory/repeated biopsy, this will help in turn reducing the fear of some patients from getting a repeated invasive procedure with its undesired consequences (TRUS biopsy). This may eventually lead to further confidence and acceptance of AS as a treatment decision among patients.

References

1. Cooperberg MR, Carroll PR, Klotz L. Active surveillance for prostate cancer: progress and promise. J Clin Oncol. 2011;29(27):3669–76.
2. Klotz L, Vesprini D, Sethukavalan P, et al. Long-term follow-up of a large active surveillance cohort of patients with prostate cancer. J Clin Oncol. 2014;33(3):272–7.
3. Sanda MG, Chen RC, Crispino T, et al. Clinically localized prostate cancer: AUA/ASTRO/SUO guideline. Risk. 2017;6:27.
4. National Comprehensive Cancer Network. Prostate Cancer (Version 4.2019). https://www.nccn.org/professionals/physician_gls/pdf/prostate.pdf. Accessed September 8, 2019
5. Bul M, Zhu X, Valdagni R, et al. Active surveillance for low-risk prostate cancer worldwide: the PRIAS study. Eur Urol. 2013;63(4):597–603.
6. Welty CJ, Cowan JE, Nguyen H, et al. Extended followup and risk factors for disease reclassification in a large active surveillance cohort for localized prostate cancer. J Urol. 2015;193(3):807–11.
7. Tosoian JJ, Trock BJ, Landis P, et al. Active surveillance program for prostate cancer: an update of the Johns Hopkins experience. J Clin Oncol. 2011;29(16):2185–90.
8. Dall'Era MA, Albertsen PC, Bangma C, et al. Active surveillance for prostate cancer: a systematic review of the literature. Eur Urol. 2012;62(6):976–83.
9. Klotz L, Lee WR, Richie MJP. Active surveillance for men with low-risk, clinically localized prostate cancer. Waltham: UpToDate; 2016.
10. Thompson I, Thrasher JB, Aus G, et al. Guideline for the management of clinically localized prostate cancer: 2007 update. J Urol. 2007;177(6):2106–31.
11. Mottet N, Bellmunt J, Bolla M, et al. EAU-ESTRO-SIOG guidelines on prostate cancer. Part 1: screening, diagnosis, and local treatment with curative intent. Eur Urol. 2017;71(4):618–29.
12. Yacoub JH, Verma S, Moulton JS, Eggener S, Oto A. Imaging-guided prostate biopsy: conventional and emerging techniques. Radiographics. 2012;32(3):819–37.
13. Choyke PL, Loeb S. Active surveillance of prostate cancer. Oncology (Williston Park). 2017;31(1):67.
14. Ahmed HU, Bosaily AE-S, Brown LC, et al. Diagnostic accuracy of multi-parametric MRI and TRUS biopsy in prostate cancer (PROMIS): a paired validating confirmatory study. Lancet. 2017;389(10071):815–22.
15. Kasivisvanathan V, Rannikko AS, Borghi M, et al. MRI-Targeted or Standard Biopsy for Prostate-Cancer Diagnosis. N Engl J Med. 2018;378(19):1767–77.
16. Siddiqui MM, Rais-Bahrami S, Turkbey B, et al. Comparison of MR/ultrasound fusion–guided biopsy with ultrasound-guided biopsy for the diagnosis of prostate cancer. JAMA. 2015;313(4):390–7.
17. Filson CP, Natarajan S, Margolis DJ, et al. Prostate cancer detection with magnetic resonance-ultrasound fusion biopsy: the role of systematic and targeted biopsies. Cancer. 2016;122(6):884–92.

18. Le JD, Stephenson S, Brugger M, et al. Magnetic resonance imaging-ultrasound fusion biopsy for prediction of final prostate pathology. J Urol. 2014;192(5):1367–73.
19. Bott S, Young M, Kellett M, Parkinson M, Contributors to the UCL Hospitals' Trust Radical Prostatectomy Database. Anterior prostate cancer: is it more difficult to diagnose? BJU Int. 2002;89(9):886–9.
20. Priester A, Natarajan S, Khoshnoodi P, et al. Magnetic resonance imaging underestimation of prostate cancer geometry: use of patient specific molds to correlate images with whole mount pathology. J Urol. 2017;197(2):320–6.
21. Schoots IG, Petrides N, Giganti F, et al. Magnetic resonance imaging in active surveillance of prostate cancer: a systematic review. Eur Urol. 2015;67(4):627–36.
22. Frye TP, George AK, Kilchevsky A, et al. Magnetic resonance imaging-transrectal ultrasound guided fusion biopsy to detect progression in patients with existing lesions on active surveillance for low and intermediate risk prostate cancer. J Urol. 2017;197(3):640–6.
23. Duffield AS, Lee TK, Miyamoto H, Carter HB, Epstein JI. Radical prostatectomy findings in patients in whom active surveillance of prostate cancer fails. J Urol. 2009;182(5):2274–9.
24. Turkbey B, Mani H, Aras O, et al. Prostate cancer: can multiparametric MR imaging help identify patients who are candidates for active surveillance? Radiology. 2013;268(1):144–52.
25. Dianat SS, Carter HB, Pienta KJ, et al. Magnetic resonance–invisible versus magnetic resonance–visible prostate cancer in active surveillance: a preliminary report on disease outcomes. Urology. 2015;85(1):147–54.
26. Elkhoury FF, Simopoulos DN, Marks LS. Targeted prostate biopsy in the era of active surveillance. Urology. 2017;112:12–9.
27. Ceylan C, Doluoglu OG, Aglamis E, Baytok O. Comparison of 8, 10, 12, 16, 20 cores prostate biopsies in the determination of prostate cancer and the importance of prostate volume. Can Urol Assoc J. 2014;8(1–2):E81.
28. Rosario DJ, Lane JA, Metcalfe C, et al. Short term outcomes of prostate biopsy in men tested for cancer by prostate specific antigen: prospective evaluation within ProtecT study. BMJ. 2012;344:d7894.
29. Nam RK, Saskin R, Lee Y, et al. Increasing hospital admission rates for urological complications after transrectal ultrasound guided prostate biopsy. J Urol. 2013;189(1):S12–8.
30. Pinkhasov GI, Lin YK, Palmerola R, et al. Complications following prostate needle biopsy requiring hospital admission or emergency department visits–experience from 1000 consecutive cases. BJU Int. 2012;110(3):369–74.
31. Lee L, Pilcher J. The role of transrectal ultrasound and biopsy in the diagnosis and management of prostate cancer. Imaging. 2008;20(2):122–30.
32. Loeb S, Vellekoop A, Ahmed HU, et al. Systematic review of complications of prostate biopsy. Eur Urol. 2013;64(6):876–92.
33. Raaijmakers R, Kirkels WJ, Roobol MJ, Wildhagen MF, Schrder FH. Complication rates and risk factors of 5802 transrectal ultrasound-guided sextant biopsies of the prostate within a population-based screening program. Urology. 2002;60(5):826–30.
34. Zaytoun OM, Anil T, Moussa AS, Jianbo L, Fareed K, Jones JS. Morbidity of prostate biopsy after simplified versus complex preparation protocols: assessment of risk factors. Urology. 2011;77(4):910–4.
35. Chowdhury R, Abbas A, Idriz S, Hoy A, Rutherford E, Smart J. Should warfarin or aspirin be stopped prior to prostate biopsy? An analysis of bleeding complications related to increasing sample number regimes. Clin Radiol. 2012;67(12):e64–70.
36. McCormack M, Duclos A, Latour M, et al. Effect of needle size on cancer detection, pain, bleeding and infection in TRUS-guided prostate biopsies: a prospective trial. Can Urol Assoc J. 2012;6(2):97.
37. Ghani KR, Dundas D, Patel U. Bleeding after transrectal ultrasonography-guided prostate biopsy: a study of 7-day morbidity after a six-, eight-and 12-core biopsy protocol. BJU Int. 2004;94(7):1014–20.
38. Berger AP, Gozzi C, Steiner H, et al. Complication rate of transrectal ultrasound guided prostate biopsy: a comparison among 3 protocols with 6, 10 and 15 cores. J Urol. 2004;171(4):1478–81.

39. Ehdaie B, Vertosick E, Spaliviero M, et al. The impact of repeat biopsies on infectious complications in men with prostate cancer on active surveillance. J Urol. 2014;191(3):660–4.
40. Batura D, Gopal Rao G. The national burden of infections after prostate biopsy in England and Wales: a wake-up call for better prevention. J Antimicrob Chemother. 2012;68(2):247–9.
41. Somford D, Hamoen E, Fütterer J, et al. The predictive value of endorectal 3 Tesla multiparametric magnetic resonance imaging for extraprostatic extension in patients with low, intermediate and high risk prostate cancer. J Urol. 2013;190(5):1728–34.
42. Villers A, Puech P, Mouton D, Leroy X, Ballereau C, Lemaitre L. Dynamic contrast enhanced, pelvic phased array magnetic resonance imaging of localized prostate cancer for predicting tumor volume: correlation with radical prostatectomy findings. J Urol. 2006;176(6):2432–7.
43. Park BH, Jang H, Song W, et al. 555 role of multiparametric 3.0 tesla magnetic resonance imaging. J Urol. 2013;189(4):e228.
44. Natarajan S, Marks LS, Margolis DJ, et al. Clinical application of a 3D ultrasound-guided prostate biopsy system. In: Paper presented at: Urologic oncology: seminars and original investigations. 2011.
45. Chang E, Jones TA, Natarajan S, et al. Value of tracking biopsy in men undergoing active surveillance of prostate cancer. J Urol. 2018;199(1):98–105.
46. Tosoian JJ, Mamawala M, Epstein JI, et al. Intermediate and longer-term outcomes from a prospective active-surveillance program for favorable-risk prostate cancer. J Clin Oncol. 2015;33(30):3379.
47. Mahran A, Turk A, Buzzy C, et al. Younger men with prostate cancer have lower risk of upgrading while on active surveillance: a meta-analysis and systematic review of the literature. Urology. 2018;121:11–8.
48. Eineluoto JT, Järvinen P, Kenttämies A, et al. Repeat multiparametric MRI in prostate cancer patients on active surveillance. PLoS One. 2017;12(12):e0189272.
49. Park BH, Jeon HG, Choo SH, et al. Role of multiparametric 3.0-T esla magnetic resonance imaging in patients with prostate cancer eligible for active surveillance. BJU Int. 2014;113(6):864–70.
50. Tan H-J, Marks LS, Hoyt MA, et al. The relationship between intolerance of uncertainty and anxiety in men on active surveillance for prostate cancer. J Urol. 2016;195(6):1724–30.
51. Anderson J, Burney S, Brooker JE, et al. Anxiety in the management of localised prostate cancer by active surveillance. BJU Int. 2014;114(S1):55–61.

A Primer on Prostate MRI for the Practicing Urologist: Update on the Current Literature

9

Kirtishri Mishra, Laura Bukavina, Amr Mahran, and Lee Ponsky

Abbreviations

AS	Active surveillance
csPCa	Clinically significant prostate cancer
mpMRI	Multi-parameteric magnetic resonance imaging
non-csPCa	Non-clinically significant prostate cancer
PCa	Prostate cancer
PI-RADS	Prostate imaging and reporting data system
PSA	Prostate specific antigen
QOL	Quality of life
TPM-biopsy	Template prostate mapping biopsy
TRUS	Transrectal ultrasound
USPSTF	United States Preventative Services Task Force

K. Mishra · L. Bukavina · A. Mahran
Urology Institute, University Hospitals Cleveland Medical Center, Cleveland, OH, USA

Case Western Reserve University School of Medicine, Cleveland, OH, USA
e-mail: kirtishri.mishra@uhhospitals.org; laura.bukavina@uhhospitals.org; amr.mahran@uhhospitals.org

L. Ponsky (✉)
Professor and Chair, Urology Institute, Leo and Charlotte Goldberg Chair of Advanced Surgical Therapies, Master Clinician in Urologic Oncology, University Hospitals Cleveland Medical Center, Case Western Reserve University School of Medicine, Cleveland, OH, USA
e-mail: Lee.Ponsky@UHhospitals.org

A. Panda et al. (eds.), *Reading MRI of the Prostate*,
https://doi.org/10.1007/978-3-319-99357-7_9

Clinical Utility of MRI

Prostate cancer (PCa) continues to be the second leading cause of cancer related death amongst men in the United States. Over the last 20 years there has been a 44% reduction in PCa related mortality, and Prostate Specific Antigen (PSA) screening is credited with a significant percentage of this reduction [1]. Recently the United States Preventative Services Task Force (USPSTF) upgraded their recommendation on screening men age 55–69 years to a Grade C, from a previous Grade D recommendation [2]. Reluctance in endorsing for PSA screening is rooted in the overtreatment of low grade PCa, which may not be a substantial contributor to overall PCa related mortality [3, 4]. In fact, of the 250,000 new diagnoses of PCa every year, only 26,120 deaths are a direct result of the disease [1]. Some may argue that we are over detecting and over treating clinically insignificant disease [4].

Current recommendations favor screening on a case-by-case basis after discussion with the patient. Recommendations against screening for PCa altogether may set us back into pre-PSA screening era; however, over detection of cancer imposes a high financial burden in an evolving cost-conscious health care system [5]. In addition to cost, elevated PSA levels trigger transrectal ultrasound guided (TRUS) biopsies, which come with their own associated risks and discomfort to patients [6, 7]. Historically, TRUS biopsies are known to under detect high-grade (clinically significant) disease while over detecting low-grade (clinically insignificant) disease [8, 9]. A potential solution to the above mentioned issues may lie in utilizing a test that can evaluate the entire prostate with high specificity, and work synergistically with PSA for detecting clinically significant PCa (csPCa). Multiparametric MRI (mpMRI) bridges this gap in the clinical domain [7, 10].

Here we provide a clinical context of multiparametric MRI (mpMRI) in a urologic setting.

Prominent Studies Associated with mpMRI

The clinical role of MRI has evolved significantly. Initially, mpMRI was used to stage post-biopsy patients for surgical planning or for radiation treatments. However, with increasing implementation of MRI, more refined data can be gleaned which allows for clinicians to discriminate between clinically significant PCa vs non-significant PCa. Currently, both European Association of Urology and National Comprehensive Cancer Network guidelines recommend prostate MRI only before repeat prostate biopsy in patients who have had previous negative biopsies, but in whom there is persistent clinical suspicion for PCa [11].

PIVOT (Prostate Cancer Intervention Versus Observation Trial)

Published in 2012 and follow-up in 2017, PIVOT has been a controversial study related to mortality for patients who underwent radical prostatectomy (RP) or observation [4, 12]. In the initial analysis, 731 patients (mean age 67 years, median

PSA 7.8 ng/mL) were randomly assigned to RP versus observation. Median follow up for the patients was 10 years. During this time, the all-cause mortality was 47.0% in the RP group and 49.9% in the observation group. The PCa specific mortality was 5.8% and 8.4% in the RP and observation groups, respectively (HR 0.63; 95% CI 0.36–1.09; $p = 0.09$). Overall, the authors concluded that the in the early era of PSA testing, there was no significant difference in the all-cause mortality and the PCa specific mortality in the RP versus observation groups [4, 12].

In the 2017 follow-up study, the authors published their data on 19.5 years of follow up (median 12.5 years). Once again, they demonstrated no significant difference in all-cause or PCa specific related mortality in the two groups. They did highlight that RP was associated with higher adverse events, but lower risk of disease and biochemical progression, and disease related symptoms [12].

The findings from the study have been challenged due to the high mortality rate in the patients reported in the PIVOT study. Froehner et al. looked at the rate of mortality in patients undergoing RP at their institution, and found that the rate of mortality reported in the PIVOT study was not reached until the age-adjusted Charlson Comorbidity index of five or higher was achieved [13]. The authors cautioned about the generalizability of the data from the PIVOT study, as they may represent high risk patients who may not have been ideal for intervention for PCa. This finding was confirmed by another study, which utilized data from Surveillance, Epidemiology, and End Results (SEER), National Caner Database (NCDB), and Prostate, Lung, Colorectal, and Ovarian cancer (PLCO) trial, which demonstrated that the patients in the PIVOT trial were significantly older than the demographics identified in this study, along with a significantly higher mortality rate [14].

The takeaway point from this study is that physicians must be well versed in the data related to pursuing surgical intervention versus observation, and if one were to take the data from PIVOT at face value, then observation is a noninferior option to surgery. In these patients, options for surveillance that yield high reliability are crucial.

ProtecT

Published in 2016, this randomized, prospective trial was the first level 1 evidence comparing the relative long-term effects on quality of life (QOL) from active surveillance (AS), surgery, and radiotherapy (RT) for patients with localized PCa [5]. A total of 1643 patients were randomized into three groups (AS, surgery, RT). The primary outcome was PCa specific mortality, and secondary outcomes were disease progression, metastases, and all-cause mortality.

The study demonstrated a 98.8% PCa specific survival rate at 10 years regardless of the randomization group, albeit the cohort was heavily (>75%) comprised of Grade 1 disease. In fact, the mortality rate was low across all three groups. In regards to the QOL outcomes, the AS group had the least deterioration in sexual function.

One of the major shortcomings of the study was that it was underpowered to evaluate the primary outcome of PCa specific mortality since the rate of mortality was lower than the rate used for the initial power calculations. In regards to the rate of metastases and disease progression, the AS group had a significantly higher rate for these secondary outcomes compared to either treatment groups; however, they did not result in increased cancer specific mortality. One reason for this may be that the data has not matured enough. Furthermore, only 44% of the original cohort in the AS group was present in the final cohort at 10 years due to crossover (either due to disease progression or from anxiety related to the disease). The ProtecT study provided high-quality evidence to incorporate AS as a routine option for patients with clinically localized PCa.

PROMIS (Diagnostic Accuracy of Multi-Parametric MRI and TRUS Biopsy in Prostate Cancer)

Published in 2017, the PROMIS study was a multi-center, paired-cohort, confirmatory study to evaluate the diagnostic accuracy of TRUS biopsy compared to mpMRI. This was compared to their reference standard of template prostate mapping biopsy (TPM-biopsy) [15]. Over the course of 3 years, 576 men underwent all three tests. The TPM-biopsy detected csPCa (defined as $\geq 4 + 3$) in 40% of the total patients, and mpMRI had a 93% sensitivity, 41% specificity, 51% positive predictive value (PPV), and 89% negative predictive value (NPV). In comparison, TRUS biopsy was significantly less sensitive (48%) with worse NPV than mpMRI (74% vs 89%). The authors of the study concluded that if mpMRI was used as a triage test, it would allow 27% of patients to avoid biopsy, and would yield a 5% decreased diagnosis of clinically insignificant cancer [15]. In other words, TRUS biopsy is inferior to mpMRI in detecting and ruling out clinically insignificant disease, while mpMRI may decrease the rate of biopsy by a quarter while also detecting less clinically insignificant cancer.

PRECISION (Prostate Evaluation for Clinically Important Disease: Sampling Using Image Guidance or Not?)

In this multicenter, randomized, noninferiority trial conducted in 2018, participants with clinical suspicion of PCa who had not undergone previous prostate biopsy were randomized to either MRI with or without targeted biopsy, and standard TRUS biopsy [16]. The study was powered for a noninferiority margin of 5%. The project was pragmatic with findings that are likely to yield practice altering evidence. In the MRI group that underwent biopsy, 38% of the patients had csPCa, while only 26% of the patients in the TRUS biopsy group had csPCa. Furthermore, fewer men in the MRI targeted group received a diagnosis of clinically insignificant cancer. Overall, this study demonstrates a superiority of MRI targeted biopsy in men with clinical risk of PCa. While there is a small chance that MRI group without biopsy may miss a small percentage of patients with csPCa that show up as PI-RADS 1 or 2 lesions, there is evidence from the Danish Cancer Registry that demonstrates that the 20-year risk of PCa specific risk of mortality after an initial negative biopsy is nearly negligible (~5%) [17].

4M (Met Prostaat MRI Meer Mans)

In this 2019, prospective, multicenter study of biopsy-naïve patients, the authors attempted to evaluate the sensitivity and specificity of pre-biopsy MRI followed by MRI guided biopsy compared to TRUS biopsy in a head-to-head study [18]. All patients underwent a pre-biopsy MRI; however, one group underwent systematic TRUS, while the other group underwent an in-gantry biopsy. They authors found that in the mpMRI pathway, csPCa was detected in 25% of the patients, while TRUS biopsy detected csPCa in 23% of the cancer. However, non-csPCa was detected only 14% of the time in mpMRI pathway, as compared to 25% in the TRUS biopsy group. While there was no statistical significance between the detection of csPCa in the two groups, this study established that mpMRI is effective at avoiding unnecessary biopsies in biopsy-naïve patients. The mpMRI pathway would avoid unnecessary biopsies in 309/626 (49%) of the patients who had non-concerning lesions on the MRI. Of these patients with non-concerning lesions, only 4% were found to have csPCa on standard biopsy at 1-year follow up. At the same time, TRUS biopsy overdetected non-csPCa in 20% of the patients [18]. This finding of missing ~5% of the cancers has been established in previous studies. Similar to previous studies, this study establishes that mpMRI is effective at avoiding unnecessary biopsies in patients with non-csPCa [17].

MRI-FIRST (Use of Prostate Systematic and Targeted Biopsy on the Basis of Multiparametric MRI in Biopsy-Naive Patients)

This 2019 study, attempts to tease out the nuances of the PRECISION study. In this multicenter, prospective, paired diagnostic study, patients with a PSA ≤20 ng/mL and stage T2c disease underwent mpMRI with a planned biopsy in <3 months [19]. The operator performing the systematic biopsy was blinded to the results of the mpMRI, and performed a standard 12 core biopsy along with two targeted biopsies of hypoechoic lesions. Subsequently, another operator performed a targeted biopsy of up to two cores of lesions that were categorized as Likert 3 or above on the likelihood of concerning lesion. Overall, the authors found that there was no difference between the systematic biopsy group versus the targeted group in detecting Grade 2 or higher cancer; however, they identified that the combination of the two methods yielded the highest likelihood of diagnosing csPCa. Therefore, while mpMRI in biopsy naïve patients may aid in identifying csPCa, it does not obviate the need for systematic biopsy [19].

This study combined with PRECISION study suggest that mpMRI can be used to triage patients for Grade 3 or higher disease; however, systematic biopsy still provides useful information on patients with Grade 2 or higher disease. It is important to point out that the MRI guided biopsies in the study were a mixture of cognitive, and fusion biopsies, but not in-gantry biopsies. The superiority of cognitive biopsy is not well established compared to a systematic biopsy [19].

Making Sense of the Data for a Urologist

Prostate cancer continues to be one of the leading causes of death in American men [2]. While we have made great progress in detecting PCa through wide-spread utilization of PSA testing, there is growing concern for over diagnosis of non-csPCa. In a 2009 study, Draisma et al. identified the range of over diagnosis to be anywhere from 23% to 42% [20]. This is one of the major limitation of PSA screening, which has drawn significant scrutiny from the national and international guidelines [2]. Over diagnosis and overtreatment not only lead to resource utilization and financial repercussions, but they also lead to patient anxiety and distress, and procedure related side-effects. One way to address this shortcoming may be to implement a screening modality that is more specific at detecting csPCa and works synergistically with PSA screening, without compromising oncologic outcomes [14, 16, 19, 21]. Based on the data provided, mpMRI may offer this adjunctive screen to improve our management of csPCa.

As demonstrated by the PROMIS study, utilization of mpMRI to triage men for prostate biopsy led to 27% decrease in primary biopsy and 5% reduction in detection of clinically insignificant cancer. In addition, the study demonstrated a possible 18% improvement in identifying clinically significant disease [15]. In addition, the PRECISION trial, further bolsters the case for routine use of mpMRI to increase detection of clinically significant cancer [16].

While there is a small chance that csPCa may be missed with utilization of pre-biopsy mpMRI, the data from the Danish Cancer Registry demonstrates that the risk of cancer specific mortatlity in this cohort is nearly negligible. On the other hand, the rate of unnecessary biopsies is reduced by 27%, and 5% of the patients avoid the diagnosis of non-csPCa, which comes with its associated benefits [17].

In an evolving health care system that is becoming increasingly cost conscious, the benefits and the risks of obtaining pre-biopsy mpMRI is a practical consideration. In the current practice, many patients undergo mpMRI only after a previous negative biopsy with persistent concern for PCa; however, this model subjects the patient to multiple procedures and related costs, along with associated side-effects and cost [2, 8]. As mpMRI becomes more mainstream, we believe that it can be performed more economically, with sustained clinical efficacy. At our institution, we offer bi-parametric MRI for $199 to patients who have been previously denied coverage from their insurance, or those who wish to benefit from the increased specificity afforded by the MRI. The clinical benefits from the bi-parametric MRI have been analyzed and our findings justify offering this option to our patients who wish to utilize it. We find that obtaining an MRI prior to biopsy can not only guide our biopsy to suspicious lesions, but more importantly, it can avoid unnecessary biopsies in patients with low grade lesions on MRI.

Ultimately, in the current landscape we endorse that patients should be assessed and counseled with all clinical variables in consideration, including patient demographics, family history, presenting symptoms, physical exam (digital rectal exam), and lab values. While no diagnostic modality is perfect, with a judicious utilization of mpMRI and targeted biopsies, we may be able to decrease the detection of clinically insignificant PCa, identify csPCa, decrease the number of unnecessary TRUS biopsies (and associated complications/cost), and devise a means for follow-up in patients undergoing AS.

References

1. Siegel RL, Miller KD, Jemal A. Cancer statistics, 2016. CA Cancer J Clin. 2016;66:7–30.
2. USPSTF Final Prostate Screening Recommendations. US Preventative Services Task Force July, 2018, July, 2018.
3. Thompson IM, Tangen CM. Prostate cancer — uncertainty and a way forward. N Engl J Med. 2012;367:270–1.
4. Wilt TJ, Brawer MK, Jones KM, et al. Radical prostatectomy versus observation for localized prostate cancer. N Engl J Med. 2012;367:203–13.
5. Hamdy FC, Donovan JL, Lane JA, et al. 10-year outcomes after monitoring, surgery, or radiotherapy for localized prostate cancer. N Engl J Med. 2016;375:1415–24.
6. Bennett HY, Roberts MJ, Doi SAR, et al. The global burden of major infectious complications following prostate biopsy. Epidemiol Infect. 2016;144:1784–91.
7. Mowatt G, Scotland G, Boachie C, et al. The diagnostic accuracy and cost-effectiveness of magnetic resonance spectroscopy and enhanced magnetic resonance imaging techniques in aiding the localisation of prostate abnormalities for biopsy: a systematic review and economic evaluation. Health Technol Assess. 2013;17:vii–xix.
8. Abraham NE, Mendhiratta N, Taneja SS. Patterns of repeat prostate biopsy in contemporary clinical practice. J Urol. 2015;193:1178–84.
9. Caverly TJ, Hayward RA, Reamer E, et al. Presentation of benefits and harms in us cancer screening and prevention guidelines: systematic review. J Natl Cancer Inst. 2016;108(6):djv436.
10. Turkbey B, Brown AM, Sankineni S, et al. Multiparametric prostate magnetic resonance imaging in the evaluation of prostate cancer. CA Cancer J Clin. 2016;66:326–36.
11. De Visschere P. Improving the diagnosis of clinically significant prostate cancer with magnetic resonance imaging. J Belg Soc Radiol. 2018;102:22. https://doi.org/10.5334/jbsr.1438. eCollection 2018.
12. Wilt TJ, Jones KM, Barry MJ, et al. Follow-up of prostatectomy versus observation for early prostate cancer. N Engl J Med. 2017;377:132–42.
13. Froehner M, Koch R, Hübler M, et al. Only <10% of patients selected for radical prostatectomy reach the competing mortality rate of the prostate cancer intervention versus observation trial (PIVOT). Eur Urol Focus. 2019;5(3):361–4.
14. Dalela D, Karabon P, Sammon J, et al. Generalizability of the prostate cancer intervention versus observation trial (PIVOT) results to contemporary north American men with prostate cancer. Eur Urol. 2017;71:511–4.
15. Ahmed HU, El-Shater Bosaily A, Brown LC, et al. Diagnostic accuracy of multi-parametric MRI and TRUS biopsy in prostate cancer (PROMIS): a paired validating confirmatory study. Lancet. 2017;389:815–22.
16. Kasivisvanathan V, Rannikko AS, Borghi M, et al. MRI-targeted or standard biopsy for prostate-cancer diagnosis. N Engl J Med. 2018;378:1767–77.
17. Klemann N, MA RÃ¸d, Helgstrand JT, et al. Risk of prostate cancer diagnosis and mortality in men with a benign initial transrectal ultrasound-guided biopsy set: a population-based study. Lancet Oncol. 2017;18:221–9.

18. van der Leest, Cornel E, Israel B, et al. Head-to-head comparison of transrectal ultrasound-guided prostate biopsy versus multiparametric prostate resonance imaging with subsequent magnetic resonance-guided biopsy in biopsy-naïve men with elevated prostate-specific antigen: a large prospective multicenter clinical study. Eur Urol. 2019;75:570–8.
19. Rouviere O, Puech P, Renard-Penna R, et al. Use of prostate systematic and targeted biopsy on the basis of multiparametric MRI in biopsy-naive patients (MRI-FIRST): a prospective, multicentre, paired diagnostic study. Lancet Oncol. 2019;20:100–9.
20. Draisma G, Etzioni R, Tsodikov A, et al. Lead time and overdiagnosis in prostate-specific antigen screening: importance of methods and context. J Natl Cancer Inst. 2009;101:374–83.
21. Gupta R, Kauffman C, Polascik T, et al. The state of prostate MRI in 2013. Oncology. 2013;27(4):262–70.

Quantitative Imaging of Prostate: Scope and Future Directions

10

Ananya Panda and Vikas Gulani

MRI is the mainstay in imaging of prostate cancer. Currently the interpretation of MRI is entirely qualitative based on visual assessment of images. While the first version of PI-RADS gave some weightage to quantitative analysis of MR spectroscopy (MRS), the second version has removed MRS and recommends visual inspection of all acquired sequences. This decision stems from the tacit understanding that quantification in MRI is technically challenging, time consuming and cannot be available or feasible at all scanners.

While quantification in MRI is difficult, there are some benefits to moving towards a more quantitative assessment. Unlike qualitative MR images which are "weighted" to provide the best signal-noise and contrast-noise ratio for visual detection of pathology, quantitative maps can give numbers that can be objective and reproducible, and have the potential to provide a degree of interpreter independence. These numbers have histologic correlates and reflect pathophysiology at a microscopic and molecular level. Potential benefits of quantification include (a) being able to non-invasively predict grades/aggressiveness of prostate cancer [1, 2] (b) differentiating prostate cancer from prostatitis and thereby avoiding unnecessary biopsies [3, 4] and (c) having objective measurements that may aid in further decision-making in patients on active surveillance [5].

As of now, diffusion weighted imaging with apparent diffusion coefficient mapping is the only truly quantitative sequence included in the multiparametric MRI protocol. While assessment is qualitative, quantification of apparent diffusion coefficient has value in diagnosis as described subsequently. Other potential methods of quantification include relaxometry; i.e. measurement of tissue relaxation times such

A. Panda
Department of Radiology, Mayo Clinic, Rochester, MN, USA
e-mail: panda.ananya@mayo.edu

V. Gulani (✉)
Fred Jenner Hodges Professor and Chair, Department of Radiology,
University of Michigan, Ann Arbor, MI, USA
e-mail: vikasgulani@med.umich.edu

A. Panda et al. (eds.), *Reading MRI of the Prostate*,
https://doi.org/10.1007/978-3-319-99357-7_10

as T1, T2 and T2*. These relaxation times reflect tissue properties and histological changes [6, 7]. Thus relaxometry may have added value to apparent diffusion coefficient mapping in differentiating grades of cancer and prostatitis from prostate cancer [4, 8]. The benefits of both apparent diffusion coefficient mapping and relaxometry are that these are non-contrast techniques and thus can potentially decrease the risks and costs of contrast administration.

DCE-MRI is another technique that can lend itself to quantification by measurement of contrast kinetics through perfusion modeling. DCE-MRI can generate numerical parameters that may be useful in baseline assessment for cancer diagnosis and longitudinal assessment for response to treatment [9, 10].

This chapter briefly describes quantitative sequences in prostate cancer imaging with examples of their clinical utility.

Quantitative Sequences

Diffusion Weighted Imaging (DWI) with Apparent Diffusion Coefficient (ADC) Mapping

In MRI, diffusion mapping in tissues almost always involves measurement of the self-diffusion of water molecules, in other words, the diffusion of water in water. A molecule on average can be thought of traveling a distance (x) in time (t) due to thermal motion, and this distance and time can be related to one another through the apparent diffusion coefficient.

At a microstructural level, water self-diffusivity is hindered by the presence of impermeable cell membranes and macromolecules. Diffusion weighted imaging probes the self-diffusivity of water by using diffusion-encoding gradients of increasing strengths and/or increased duration, the combined effect of which is denoted by the term b-value. Images acquired with greater diffusion sensitivity (higher b values) show more diffusion-related signal decay. The larger the diffusivity of a substance or tissue, the more the signal decays, and the darker that tissue will appear on diffusion-weighted images. Modeling the signal decay between two or more different b-values gives the 'apparent diffusion coefficient". The term "apparent" is used to acknowledge the fact that the signal decay used to calculate the diffusivity in MRI contains contributions from all sources of motion, not just pure diffusion. For diffusion weighted imaging in the prostate, typically high b-values are used (>800 s/mm^2 and up to 1400 or 2000 s/mm^2). In the calculation of the apparent diffusion coefficient, the signal decay is assumed to be monoexponential and it is also assumed that all diffusion is taking place in a single, well-mixed compartment. These assumptions are never fully true in tissue. The calculation of the apparent diffusivity includes the additional signal decay that occurs due to diffusion of water within capillaries. However, using multiple b-values less than 200 s/mm^2, and biexponential models, it is also possible to get additional parameters which give information about microperfusion within a voxel. This technique is called intravoxel incoherent motion (IVIM) [11]. There is extensive ongoing research exploring non-monoexponential, multicompartmental diffusion, both regarding IVIM and also utilizing very high b-value imaging to separate intracellular and extracellular contributions to the apparent diffusivity as seen by MRI. A detailed discussion of these issues is beyond the scope of this book.

Apparent diffusion coefficient mapping allows the measurement of the mobility of water molecules in water at a cellular level and is profoundly affected by tissue cellularity and tissue organization. Studies have shown that the apparent diffusion coefficients are significantly different between prostate cancers and normal peripheral zone and normal transition zone [3, 12, 13]. In addition, apparent diffusion coefficient values correlate inversely with tumor grade [1, 12, 14, 15]. The clinical utility and ranges of apparent diffusion coefficients values have been described in more detail subsequently.

DCE-MRI with Perfusion Modeling

In DCE-MRI, perfusion parameters can be obtained by administering intravenous gadolinium-based contrast agent, acquiring multiple T1 weighted images at a very high temporal resolution (<10 s/volume) for at least 2–3 min, and performing pharmacokinetic modeling to extract quantitative parameters. The most common model used is a compartmental model with a single tissue compartment [16]. This assumes exchange of contrast material between the intravascular space and extravascular extracellular space as depicted in Fig. 10.1. The parameters obtained include:

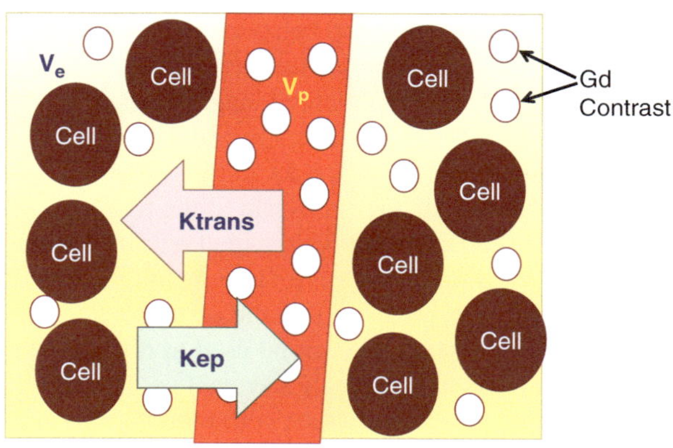

Fig. 10.1 A pictorial representation of the extended Toft's pharmacokinetic model used in DCE-MRI. The red rectangle represents blood capillary while yellow area represents extravascular space containing cells and interstitial tissue. Ktrans (pink arrow) refers to the rate of influx of gadolinium contrast (white circles) from the vascular space to extracellular space while Kep (green arrow) refers to the rate of efflux of contrast from extracellular space back into the vascular space. Ve: refers to the volume of extracellular space while Vp refers to plasma volume

(a) Ktrans: rate of influx of contrast from vascular space to extracellular space (measure of permeability)
(b) Kep: rate of efflux of contrast from extracellular space to vascular space
(c) Ve: interstitial volume/ volume of extracellular space
(d) Vp: plasma volume

Studies have shown that Ktrans and Kep are higher in tumors than normal peripheral zone [17]. In addition, Ktrans is significantly higher in intermediate and high-grade prostate cancers compared to low-grade cancers [18, 19]. However the role of quantitative DCE-MRI metrics in transition zone cancers is less clear, and this is reflected in the fact that DCE imaging is not included for assessment of the transition zone in PI-RADS version 2 [20, 21].

Perfusion modeling is complex; the metrics obtained depend on the pharmacokinetic model used, selection of arterial input function, contrast dose, contrast injection rate, temporal resolution, etc. [22, 23]. This has led to variability that limits the general quantitative applicability of this technique and limits comparison between different studies. Moreover, quantitative DCE-MRI metrics have a lower overall diagnostic performance and lower additive value as compared to apparent diffusion coefficient mapping. Hence, quantitative DCE-MRI criteria may presently be more suitable for longitudinal studies performing DCE-MRI with the same technique or for detection of tumor recurrence rather than for primary detection or characterization of prostate cancer [24].

Relaxometry

Relaxometry is the measurement of tissue relaxation times, most commonly T1, T2 and T2*. These relaxation times reflect the behavior of proton spins in the presence of externally applied radiofrequency pulses used to generate MR signals. T1 relaxation time is the time taken for the longitudinal magnetization to recover two-thirds of its initial value whereas T2 is the time taken for the transverse magnetization component to decay to about one-third of its initial value. T1 and T2 represent MR-specific tissue properties, which are intrinsic to the tissue under evaluation. In addition, T2* is another derived tissue property which reflects the effective T2 decay in the presence of local field inhomogeneities and susceptibility effects. Measurement of relaxation times are useful as they can provide objective and direct quantitative information about tissues in a voxel and can be used to differentiate various tissue entities. Previous studies have shown that T2 as well as T2* shortening is seen in prostate cancer as compared to normal tissues with more aggressive cancers having shorter T2 or T2* relaxation times compared to low-grade (Gleason score $3 + 3 = 6$) cancers [7, 25–28].

However, relaxometry can be quite challenging and time consuming and conventional mapping sequences typically measure only one tissue property at a time (either T1 or T2) and thus are not routinely used in clinical practice. More recently, a new approach to relaxometry was described, and termed MR Fingerprinting (MRF), which allows simultaneous mapping of T1 and T2 relaxation times in a time-efficient manner and is highly robust, repeatable and reproducible [29]. In MR Fingerprinting, instead of using preset MR system parameters to obtain either T1 and T2 weighted images, these system parameters are allowed to vary in a pseudorandom manner to generate a dictionary of unique signal evolutions, for each combination of tissue properties of interest. The signal evolutions from individual voxels are compared with the dictionary by a pattern-matching process on a voxel-by-voxel basis to generate perfectly co-registered T1 and T2 maps that provide both anatomic and quantitative information [30, 31]. Preliminary results have shown that MR Fingerprinting relaxometry in combination with apparent diffusion coefficient mapping can differentiate between normal peripheral zone and prostate cancer and prostatitis in the peripheral zone [4], Subsequently this technique has been further explored for transition zone and validated in combination with targeted biopsies as described subsequently [32, 33]. Synthetic MRI is another technique that can allow simultaneous estimation of T1 and T2 relaxation times. At present, there is a paucity of robust histologic validation studies using prostate synthetic MRI.

Clinical Utility of Quantitative Assessment: Present Evidence and Future Directions

Predicting Aggressiveness of Prostate Cancer

Clinically, it is important to differentiate low-grade cancers (Gleason score 3 + 3 = 6) from intermediate and high-grade cancers (Gleason scores 7 and above) as low-grade cancers are considered clinically insignificant and do not require immediate treatment. Quantitative MRI has shown to be useful in this scenario. Clinically significant prostate cancer is histologically characterized by increased cellularity, increased nuclear percentage area and decreased lumen area. The combined effect of these histological changes leads to decrease in diffusivity of water, which is reflected by lower apparent diffusion coefficient values and shorter T2 and $T2^*$ relaxation times in more aggressive cancers [8, 25, 26]. On the other hand, low-grade tumors and histologically sparse tumors have intermixed normal tissue and thus the apparent diffusion coefficients and T2 values in these tumors are similar to normal prostate tissue [34].

Different studies have explored the range of apparent diffusion coefficient values for prostate cancer grades at both 1.5 T and 3 T MR systems. In a study by Bittencourt, et al. [2] performed at 1.5 T, peripheral zone low-grade tumors had a mean apparent diffusion coefficient range of 0. 91 × 10^{-3} mm/s^2 while intermediate/high grade tumors (Gleason score 7 and above) had a mean apparent diffusion coefficient of

0.71×10^{-3} mm/s^2 with an area under curve of = 0.82 for differentiating peripheral zone tumors. In another study at 3 T MRI system, the discriminatory performance of apparent diffusion coefficient was 0.90 in differentiation of low from intermediate/high grade tumors. Multiple studies have shown that the median apparent diffusion coefficient for low-grade cancers is $1.1–1.3 \times 10^{-3}$ mm/s^2, intermediate grade cancers is $0.87–1.01 \times 10^{-3}$ mm/s^2 and high grade cancers was $0.69–0.94 \times 10^{-3}$ mm/s^2. Since there is an overlap in apparent diffusion coefficient values, most radiologists usually use a cut-off of $0.75–0.90 \times 10^{-3}$ mm/s^2 to differentiate clinically significant cancers from insignificant/low-grade cancers.

Combining relaxometry with apparent diffusion coefficient mapping improves the overall area under curve for determining cancer aggressiveness. A recent study using MR Fingerprinting relaxometry with TRUS biopsy correlation in peripheral zone tumors showed that discriminatory area under curves for both MR

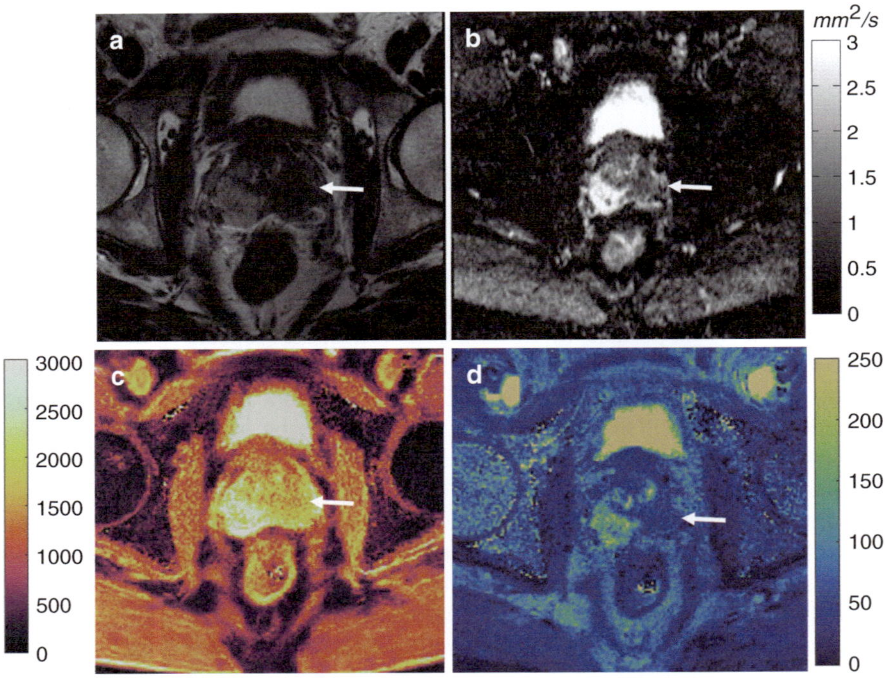

Fig. 10.2 T2 weighted image (**a**), apparent diffusion coefficient map (**b**), MR Fingerprinting T1 color map (**c**) and MR Fingerprinting T2 color map (**d**) of a patient with biopsy –proven case of high-grade prostate cancer (Gleason score 4 + 4 = 8). T2 weighted image shows a large dark lesion in left peripheral zone with extracapsular extension (arrow, **a**). The apparent diffusion coefficient value was $0.42 \pm 0.05 \times 10^{-3}$ mm^2/s (**b**), T1 was 1690 ± 270 ms and T2 was 47 ± 18 ms, all consistent with ranges of values described for high-grade prostate cancer in literature

Fingerprinting-T2 and apparent diffusion coefficient individually were 0.77; combining these two properties improved the area under curve to 0.83 for differentiating low-grade from intermediate to high-grade peripheral zone prostate cancers [4] (Fig. 10.2). Moreover, using targeted biopsy validation, the combination of MR Fingerprinting-T2 values and apparent diffusion coefficients had an even higher discriminatory ability with area under curve of 0.91 [33]. Since both MR Fingerprinting based- T2 mapping and apparent diffusion coefficient have comparable diagnostic discriminatory performance, T2 mapping can be potentially helpful when apparent diffusion coefficient maps are distorted due to susceptibility artefacts.

The significance of apparent diffusion coefficient mapping in transition zone and central zone tumors is less clear as compared to peripheral zone tumors [35, 36]. In a study by Jung et al. [37], the apparent diffusion coefficient values in benign glandular hyperplasia (1.44–1.49 × 10^{-3} mm/s^2) was significantly higher than all prostate cancers whereas apparent diffusion coefficient values of stromal hyperplasia (1.1 × 10^{-3} mm/s^2) were only significantly higher than clinically significant cancers (0.70–0.99 × 10^{-3} mm/s^2). Thus, there is an overlap between apparent diffusion coefficient values of benign stromal nodules and low-grade cancer. The role of relaxometry in predicting grades of transition zone tumors is less defined as compared to peripheral zone. However, MR Fingerprinting relaxometry with co-registered T1 and T2 maps has been shown to provide additional discriminatory information in differentiating transition zone cancers from prostatitis and benign nodules [32].

Differentiating Prostatitis from Prostate Cancer

Apart from detection and characterization of prostate cancer, another objective of prostate MRI is to reduce the number of false positives and reduce unnecessary biopsies. Prostatitis is a common cause of false positive reads on MRI based on T2 weighted images alone. Apparent diffusion coefficient mapping alone has moderate discriminatory value in differentiating between prostatitis and prostate cancer with are under curves ranging from 0.62–0.84 [35, 38, 39]. The median apparent diffusion coefficient values for prostatitis ranges from 0.91–1.37 × 10^{-3} mm/s^2 and does overlap with apparent diffusion coefficient values in low-grade cancers [3, 4].

However, MR Fingerprinting relaxometry additionally revealed that, the mean T1 and T2 relaxation times in prostatitis were significantly higher compared to cancer in both peripheral and transition zones and thus may be used in combination with apparent diffusion coefficient mapping to improve differentiation between the two entities [32, 33]. Despite both prostatitis and cancer looking similar on T2 weighted images, the T1 relaxation time could specifically help differentiate between the two entities in the transition zone [32]. (Fig. 10.3).

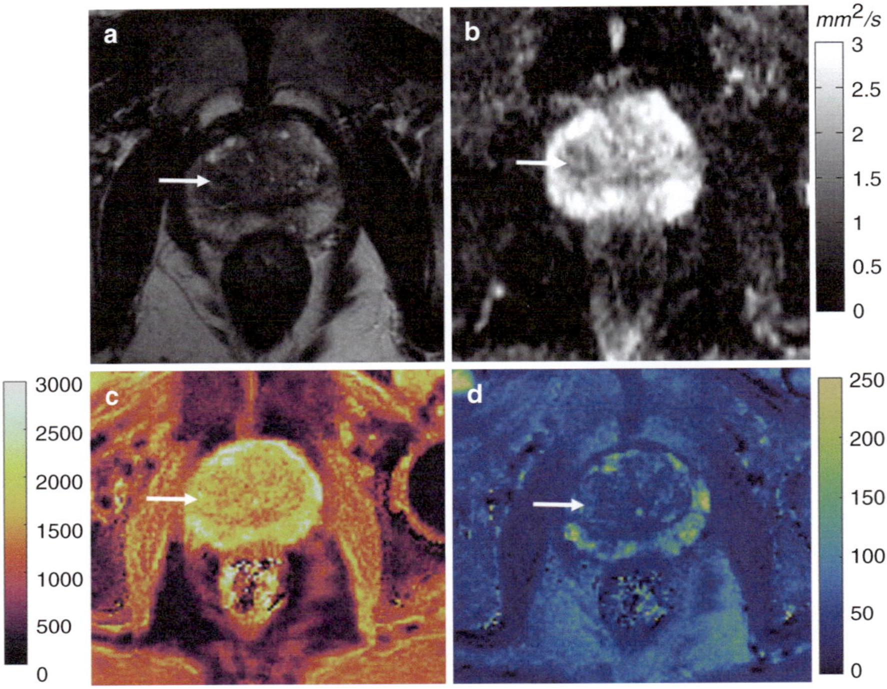

Fig. 10.3 T2 weighted image (**a**), apparent diffusion coefficient map (**b**), MR Fingerprinting T1 color map (**c**) and MR Fingerprinting T2 color map (**d**) of a patient with biopsy—proven case of prostatitis. T2 weighted image shows a focal lesion in left anterior transition zone with low signal intensity and lobulated margins (arrow, **a**). The lesion also had a low apparent diffusion coefficient (0.87×10^{-3} mm^2/s) and was reported as PI-RADS 3. MR Fingerprinting maps showed that T1 was 1690 ± 170 ms and T2 was 63 ± 14 ms and T1 value was consistent with that of non-cancerous lesions

Follow-up Assessment in Patients on Active Surveillance

MRI plays an important role in selecting patients for active surveillance and for reassessment of disease status. Quantitative criteria may be useful in determining disease progression on follow-up MRIs, thereby decreasing the number of subsequent restaging biopsies. In a study by Felker et al. [40], the predictive area under curve of a model based on clinical criteria alone was 0.87 and combining this with serial multiparametric MRI data increased the area under curve to 0.91 in non-invasively predicting disease progression [40]. Morgan, et al. [5], longitudinally tracked the changes in apparent diffusion coefficient and tumor volume in patients on active surveillance and found that change in apparent diffusion coefficient was

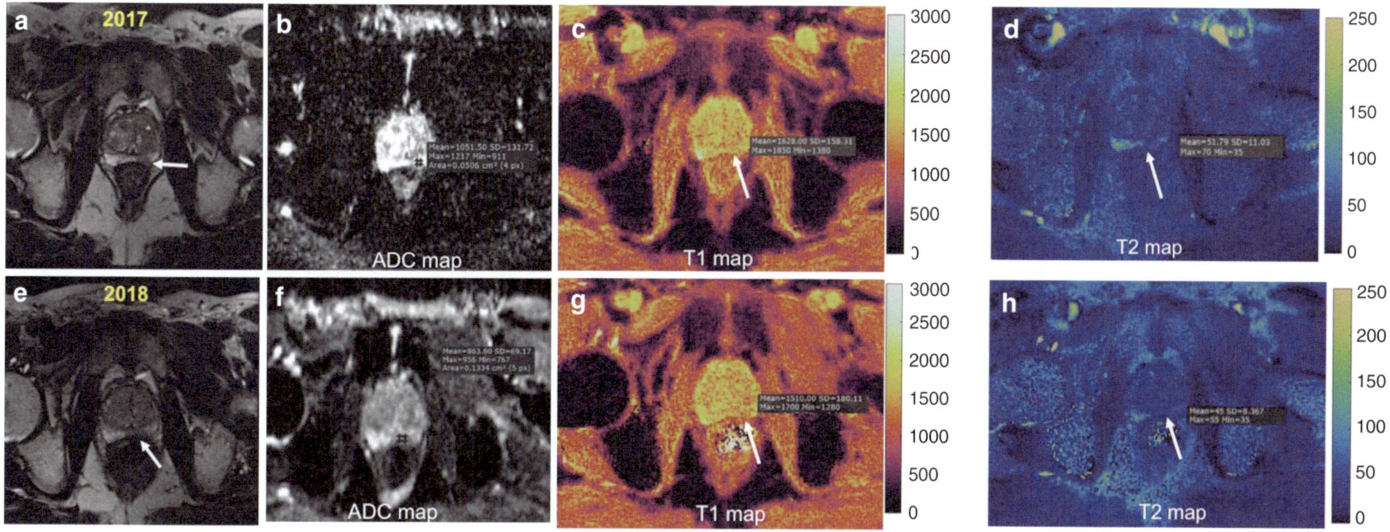

Fig. 10.4 Serial T2 weighted image (**a**, **e**), apparent diffusion coefficient map (**b**, **f**), MR Fingerprinting T1 color map (**c**, **g**) and MR Fingerprinting T2 color map (**d**, **h**) of a patient with biopsy –proven case of Gleason score 3 + 3 = 6 cancer on active surveillance. Imaging was repeated after 1 year. Both the T2 weighted images obtained in 2017 and 2018 show an ill-defined dark lesion in left posteromedial peripheral zone (arrows **a**, **d**). While the lesion looks qualitatively/visually similar, there is decrease in apparent diffusion coefficient values (2017: $1.05 \pm 0.13 \times 10^{-3}$ mm^2/s; 2018: $0.86 \pm 0.07 \times 10^{-3}$ mm^2/s), decrease in T1 (2017: 1630 ± 160 ms, 2018: 1510 ± 180 ms) and relatively similar T2 values (2017: 52 ± 11 ms, 2018: 45 ± 8 ms). Repeat biopsy showed Gleason score 3 + 4 = 7 cancer

significantly different in patients with tumor growth versus those without ($p = 0.0005$) and the percentage change in tumor was negatively correlated with percentage change in apparent diffusion coefficient ($r = -0.31$, $p = 0.0001$) (Fig. 10.4).

Summary

Apparent diffusion coefficient mapping and relaxometry both provide windows of opportunities in objective assessment and longitudinal follow-up in prostate cancer. While diffusion weighted imaging with apparent diffusion coefficient mapping is already a standard of care, relaxometry is a relatively new development in prostate imaging. In the future, combining quantitative assessment with multiparametric MRI may reduce the number of biopsies or avoid unnecessary biopsies altogether, or allow patients to be followed with more confidence in active surveillance protocols.

References

1. Vargas HA, Akin O, Franiel T, Mazaheri Y, Zheng J, Moskowitz C, et al. Diffusion-weighted endorectal MR imaging at 3 T for prostate cancer: tumor detection and assessment of aggressiveness. Radiology. 2011;259(3):775–84.
2. Bittencourt LK, Barentsz JO, Miranda LCD, de Gasparetto EL. Prostate MRI: diffusion-weighted imaging at 1.5T correlates better with prostatectomy Gleason grades than TRUS-guided biopsies in peripheral zone tumours. Eur Radiol. 2012;22(2):468–75.
3. Nagel KNA, Schouten MG, Hambrock T, Litjens GJS, Hoeks CMA, ten Haken B, et al. Differentiation of prostatitis and prostate cancer by using diffusion-weighted MR imaging and MR-guided biopsy at 3 T. Radiology. 2013;267(1):164–72.
4. Yu AC, Badve C, Ponsky LE, Pahwa S, Dastmalchian S, Rogers M, et al. Development of a combined MR fingerprinting and diffusion examination for prostate cancer. Radiology. 2017;283(3):729–38.
5. Morgan VA, Parker C, MacDonald A, Thomas K, de Souza NM. Monitoring tumor volume in patients with prostate cancer undergoing active surveillance: is MRI apparent diffusion coefficient indicative of tumor growth? AJR Am J Roentgenol. 2017;209(3):620–8.
6. Gibbs P, Liney GP, Pickles MD, Zelhof B, Rodrigues G, Turnbull LW. Correlation of ADC and T2 measurements with cell density in prostate cancer at 3.0 tesla. Investig Radiol. 2009;44(9):572–6.
7. Langer DL, van der Kwast TH, Evans AJ, Plotkin A, Trachtenberg J, Wilson BC, et al. Prostate tissue composition and mr measurements: investigating the relationships between ADC, T2, Ktrans, ve, and corresponding histologic features. Radiology. 2010;255(2):485–94.
8. Wu L-M, Zhou B, Lu Q, Suo S-T, Liu Q, Hu J, et al. T2* relaxation time in the detection and assessment of aggressiveness of peripheral zone cancer in comparison with diffusion-weighted imaging. Clin Radiol. 2016;71(4):356–62.
9. Verma S, Turkbey B, Muradyan N, Rajesh A, Cornud F, Haider MA, et al. Overview of dynamic contrast-enhanced MRI in prostate cancer diagnosis and management. AJR Am J Roentgenol. 2012;198(6):1277–88.
10. Hötker AM, Mazaheri Y, Aras Ö, Zheng J, Moskowitz CS, Gondo T, et al. Assessment of prostate cancer aggressiveness by use of the combination of quantitative DWI and dynamic contrast-enhanced MRI. AJR Am J Roentgenol. 2016;206(4):756–63.

11. Iima M, Le Bihan D. Clinical intravoxel incoherent motion and diffusion MR imaging: past, present, and future. Radiology. 2015;278(1):13–32.
12. Tamada T, Sone T, Jo Y, Toshimitsu S, Yamashita T, Yamamoto A, et al. Apparent diffusion coefficient values in peripheral and transition zones of the prostate: comparison between normal and malignant prostatic tissues and correlation with histologic grade. J Magn Reson Imaging. 2008;28(3):720–6.
13. Kim CK, Park BK, Han JJ, Kang TW, Lee HM. Diffusion-weighted imaging of the prostate at 3 T for differentiation of malignant and benign tissue in transition and peripheral zones: preliminary results. J Comput Assist Tomogr. 2007;31(3):449–54.
14. deSouza NM, Riches SF, Vanas NJ, Morgan VA, Ashley SA, Fisher C, et al. Diffusion-weighted magnetic resonance imaging: a potential non-invasive marker of tumour aggressiveness in localized prostate cancer. Clin Radiol. 2008;63(7):774–82.
15. Tamada T, Prabhu V, Li J, Babb JS, Taneja SS, Rosenkrantz AB. Prostate cancer: diffusion-weighted MR imaging for detection and assessment of aggressiveness-comparison between conventional and kurtosis models. Radiology. 2017;284(1):100–8.
16. Sourbron S. Technical aspects of MR perfusion. Eur J Radiol. 2010;76(3):304–13.
17. Gao P, Shi C, Zhao L, Zhou Q, Luo L. Differential diagnosis of prostate cancer and noncancerous tissue in the peripheral zone and central gland using the quantitative parameters of DCE-MRI. Medicine (Baltimore). 2016;95(52):e5715. Available from: https://www.ncbi.nlm.nih.gov/pmc/articles/PMC5207570/.
18. Vos EK, Litjens GJS, Kobus T, Hambrock T, Hulsbergen-van de Kaa CA, Barentsz JO, et al. Assessment of prostate cancer aggressiveness using dynamic contrast-enhanced magnetic resonance imaging at 3 T. Eur Urol. 2013;64(3):448–55.
19. Ocak I, Bernardo M, Metzger G, Barrett T, Pinto P, Albert PS, et al. Dynamic contrast-enhanced MRI of prostate cancer at 3 T: a study of pharmacokinetic parameters. AJR Am J Roentgenol. 2007;189(4):849.
20. Hoeks CMA, Hambrock T, Yakar D, Hulsbergen–van de Kaa CA, Feuth T, Witjes JA, et al. Transition zone prostate cancer: detection and localization with 3-T multiparametric MR imaging. Radiology. 2013;266(1):207–17.
21. Chesnais AL, Niaf E, Bratan F, Mège-Lechevallier F, Roche S, Rabilloud M, et al. Differentiation of transitional zone prostate cancer from benign hyperplasia nodules: evaluation of discriminant criteria at multiparametric MRI. Clin Radiol. 2013;68(6):e323–30.
22. Othman AE, Falkner F, Kessler D-E, Martirosian P, Weiss J, Kruck S, et al. Comparison of different population-averaged arterial-input-functions in dynamic contrast-enhanced MRI of the prostate: effects on pharmacokinetic parameters and their diagnostic performance. Magn Reson Imaging. 2016;34(4):496–501.
23. Ream JM, Doshi AM, Dunst D, Parikh N, Kong MX, Babb JS, et al. Dynamic contrast-enhanced MRI of the prostate: an intraindividual assessment of the effect of temporal resolution on qualitative detection and quantitative analysis of histopathologically proven prostate cancer. J Magn Reson Imaging. 2017;45(5):1464–75.
24. Low RN, Fuller DB, Muradyan N. Dynamic gadolinium-enhanced perfusion MRI of prostate cancer: assessment of response to hypofractionated robotic stereotactic body radiation therapy. AJR Am J Roentgenol. 2011;197(4):907–15.
25. Gibbs P, Tozer DJ, Liney GP, Turnbull LW. Comparison of quantitative T2 mapping and diffusion-weighted imaging in the normal and pathologic prostate. Magn Reson Med. 2001;46(6):1054–8.
26. Langer DL, van der Kwast TH, Evans AJ, Trachtenberg J, Wilson BC, Haider MA. Prostate cancer detection with multi-parametric MRI: logistic regression analysis of quantitative T2, diffusion-weighted imaging, and dynamic contrast-enhanced MRI. J Magn Reson Imaging. 2009;30(2):327–34.
27. Wu L-M, Chen X-X, Xuan H-Q, Liu Q, Suo S-T, Hu J, et al. Feasibility and preliminary experience of quantitative T2* mapping at 3.0 T for detection and assessment of aggressiveness of prostate cancer. Acad Radiol. 2014;21(8):1020–6.

28. Wu L-M, Zhao Z-Z, Chen X-X, Lu Q, Suo S-T, Liu Q, et al. Comparison of T2* mapping with diffusion-weighted imaging in the characterization of low-grade vs intermediate-grade and high-grade prostate cancer. Br J Radiol. 2016;89(1063):20151076.
29. Lo W, et al. Multicenter repeatability and reproducibility of MR Fingerprinting [Internet]. Joint Annual Meeting ISMRM-ESMRMB; 2018 Jun 19; Paris, France. Available from: http://cds.ismrm.org/protected/18MPresentations/abstracts/4503.html.
30. Ma D, Gulani V, Seiberlich N, Liu K, Sunshine JL, Duerk JL, et al. Magnetic resonance fingerprinting. Nature. 2013;495(7440):187–92.
31. Jiang Y, Ma D, Seiberlich N, Gulani V, Griswold MA. MR fingerprinting using fast imaging with steady state precession (FISP) with spiral readout. Magn Reson Med. 2015;74(6):1621–31.
32. Panda A, Obmann VC, Lo WC, Margevicius S, Jiang Y, Schluchter M, et al. MR Fingerprinting and ADC Mapping for Characterization of Lesions in the Transition Zone of the Prostate Gland. Radiology. 2019;292(3):685–94. https://doi.org/10.1148/radiol.2019181705.
33. Panda A, O'Connor G, Lo WC, Jiang Y, Margevicius S, Schluchter M, Ponsky LE, Gulani V. Targeted biopsy validation of peripheral zone prostate cancer characterization with magnetic resonance fingerprinting and diffusion mapping. Investig Radiol. 2019;54(8):485–93. https://doi.org/10.1097/RLI.0000000000000569. PMID: 30985480.
34. Langer DL, van der Kwast TH, Evans AJ, Sun L, Yaffe MJ, Trachtenberg J, et al. Intermixed normal tissue within prostate cancer: effect on MR imaging measurements of apparent diffusion coefficient and T2—sparse versus dense cancers. Radiology. 2008;249(3):900–8.
35. Hoeks CMA, Vos EK, Bomers JGR, Barentsz JO, Hulsbergen-van de Kaa CA, Scheenen TW. Diffusion-weighted magnetic resonance imaging in the prostate transition zone: histopathological validation using magnetic resonance–guided biopsy specimens. Investig Radiol. 2013;48(10):693–701.
36. Kim JH, Kim JK, Park B-W, Kim N, Cho K-S. Apparent diffusion coefficient: prostate cancer versus noncancerous tissue according to anatomical region. J Magn Reson Imaging. 2008;28(5):1173–9.
37. Jung SI, Donati OF, Vargas HA, Goldman D, Hricak H, Akin O. Transition zone prostate cancer: incremental value of diffusion-weighted endorectal MR imaging in tumor detection and assessment of aggressiveness. Radiology. 2013;269(2):493–503.
38. Simpkin CJ, Morgan VA, Giles SL, Riches SF, Parker C, de Souza NM. Relationship between T2 relaxation and apparent diffusion coefficient in malignant and non-malignant prostate regions and the effect of peripheral zone fractional volume. Br J Radiol. 2013;86(1024):20120469.
39. Esen M, Onur MR, Akpolat N, Orhan I, Kocakoc E. Utility of ADC measurement on diffusion-weighted MRI in differentiation of prostate cancer, normal prostate and prostatitis. Quant Imaging Med Surg. 2013;3(4):210–6.
40. Felker ER, Wu J, Natarajan S, Margolis DJ, Raman SS, Huang J, et al. Serial magnetic resonance imaging in active surveillance of prostate cancer: incremental value. J Urol. 2016;195(5):1421–7.

Index

A. Panda et al. (eds.), *Reading MRI of the Prostate*,
https://doi.org/10.1007/978-3-319-99357-7

MIX
Papier aus verantwortungsvollen Quellen
Paper from responsible sources
FSC® C105338

If you have any concerns about our products,
you can contact us on
ProductSafety@springernature.com

In case Publisher is established outside the EU,
the EU authorized representative is:
Springer Nature Customer Service Center GmbH
Europaplatz 3, 69115 Heidelberg, Germany

Printed by Libri Plureos GmbH
in Hamburg, Germany